Home Care

৯৯৯Home Care Living with Dying

Edited by
> **Elizabeth R. Prichard,**
> **Jean Collard,**
> **Janet Starr,**
> **Josephine A. Lockwood,**
> **Austin H. Kutscher, and**
> **Irene B. Seeland**

With the Editorial Assistance of
> **Lillian G. Kutscher**

Columbia University Press · New York · 1979

Columbia University Press
New York   Guildford, Surrey

Copyright © 1979 by Columbia University Press
All Rights Reserved
Printed in the United States of America

Library of Congress Cataloging in Publication Data

Main entry under title:

Home care: living with dying.

    Includes bibliographies and index.
    1. Terminal care.   2. Home care services.
3. Death—Psychological aspects.   4. Cancer
patients—Home care.   I. Prichard, Elizabeth R.
R728.8.H65   362.1′4   78–21983
ISBN 0–231–04258-2

⁂ Acknowledgment

The editors wish to acknowledge the support and encouragement of the Foundation of Thanatology in the preparation of this volume. All royalties from the sale of this book are assigned to the Foundation of Thanatology, a tax exempt, not for profit, public research and educational foundation.

Thanatology, a new subspecialty of medicine, is involved in scientific and humanistic inquiries and the application of the knowledge derived therefrom to the subjects of the psychological aspects of dying; reactions to loss, death, and grief; and recovery from bereavement.

The Foundation of Thanatology is dedicated to advancing the cause of enlightened health care for the terminally ill patient and his family. The Foundation's orientation is a positive one based on the philosophy of fostering a more mature acceptance and understanding of death and the problems of grief and the more effective and humane management and treatment of the dying patient and his bereaved family members.

⌇⌇⌇ Contents

Part III. Home Care Services

Part IV. Community Resources and Responsibilities

Part V. Research Needs

Part VI. From Life to Death

≈≈≈Foreword

The Totality of Care— from Birth to Death

Samuel C. Klagsbrun

We have to go back to our roots in thanatology, whether from a research or a clinical point of view. My own personal roots relate closely to my grandmother. She knew very well what home care was all about. She did not trust hospitals; she said that hospitals were places where one went to die. Perhaps she was right. She was also the person who used to take an aspirin for her occasional headaches, cutting it in half and then biting off a quarter. She would feel much, much better after she spit out the quarter. If a paranoid flavor tinges my feelings about institutional health care, it is clear from whence it comes. Unfortunately, my grandmother died in a hospital a number of years ago, much against her will. If we had been wise in those years, we might have spared her that experience.

Home care is a traditional way of thinking about dealing with illness; it has become untraditional only in modern times. We have paid a high price for forgetting about home care for so many years.

In medical school I was brought back sharply to the ideas prevalent in what old-fashioned doctors took for granted—that is, what one does in a home can probably be far better than what one could do in a hospital setting. For example, we spent our obstetric rotation in the Maxwell Street Dispensary in the middle of the south side of Chicago. We said goodbye to our families, took some change of underwear, and disappeared for two weeks. We lived in the middle of the south side in a very old, wooden-frame house that had a large switchboard downstairs. That was the only nice thing it had; the rest of it was incredible. That switchboard took calls in from women who chose to have the Maxwell Street Dispensary doctors—we were all junior medical students—come to their homes and deliver their babies at home. Since we were "expert" obstetricians, we took our *Merck Manuals* in one hand and a bottle of saline in the other. (We were not allowed to dispense drugs, because we were not licensed physicians.) In a dire emergency the only thing we could do was prevent shock. Of course, we were allowed to take a bottle of saline and go into their homes and live with the people who had called on us for the labor and the delivery. We were expected to stay there for a couple of hours afterward, at the end of which, if everything was all right, we would return to the dispensary, grab a couple of hours' sleep, and then answer the next call. We did this for two weeks, around the clock, day in, day out.

That was the most exhilarating experience of my entire medical school career. I still go back to that period of time and think about home care under those circumstances. The south side of Chicago is probably the equivalent of the Harlem geographical area in New York City. Originally, we worried about everything from safety to sanitation. We were called into some of the nicest homes that I have ever had the privilege of seeing. The people simply took us for granted as persons who belonged in the area, who did a good job, and who were committed.

The qualities that got us through had nothing to do with the practice of sophisticated medicine. We were not good doctors, in the sense of having good medical knowledge. What got us through—and it is fascinating to see the physical results of those experiences—was the commitment, which is the kind of thing, I think, that can take place only at home in its most nearly unique form. One can be committed to a person in the hospital, but one has a culture to work *against* in the hospital. One has a culture to work *with* in the home setting. For example, during the two weeks in the obstetrical rotation in the hospital, I delivered a number of babies and had a number of cervical tears requiring stitches. *No* delivery that I did in the home required a single stitch!

What were the other differences? I was called in at some point when the woman was in labor. She trusted me because *she* was the one who had called me and she knew that it was known in the area that I would go out, I would sit, and I had no other responsibility except her. There was nothing else to bother me—no television, no telephones (most of the homes did not have any)—I just sat there and talked. Sometimes in a very complicated, prolonged labor I might spend 18 hours with a woman. Sometimes I might spend only four hours. The point is I was there with that person, alone, with nothing else except who I was as a human being because what was in my bag was nothing, and she knew it and I knew it.

There was a backup system available in case either the patient or we got into trouble. Sometimes it was hard to tell who was more in need. Fortunately, I did not have to rely on the backup system. Not a single tear occurred and the babies were healthy. It is a marvelous, thrilling experience to have that kind of opportunity to do home care.

I am stressing birth even in this context of thanatology (and many aspects of birth have thanatologic dimensions) to draw on other resources that have less to do with death and dying as concepts applicable to the issue of home care and death and dying, which is not an isolated phenomenon. It is part of *total care,* whether one is talking about birth, psychiatry, day hospitalization, or home visits. There is no difference.

While doing home care nursing through the St. Christopher's Hospice in London, I went on rounds with the staff and learned a great deal about the continuity of care available in a home setting, a continuity that is difficult to come by in the hospital settings, where staff, residents, and interns constantly rotate, change identities, and shift to different floors, having different roommates every few days.

At St. Luke's Hospital (New York City), in the Psychiatric Day Hospital, we made it part of our job to see every single one of our Day Hospital patients in a home setting at some point within the first two weeks of admission. This was done simply to gather information. It is the same as in group therapy. One is a different person, or more properly stated, a different side of one's personality gets expressed and is visible when one is at home. To have a proper understanding of the total picture, of the total person, it is crucial to see that person in a home setting.

What is required for the success of a home care program? We must offer ourselves as backup systems for the relatives at home. If a wife of a sick husband feels that she is being backed up, she will be a superb person in terms of caring for her husband. If she feels that she is going to be abandoned after the visit, that there is no possibility of reaching the physician or others in an emergency, she will very quickly feel undermined and will not be able to take care of her husband as well as she might under other circumstances. So the concept of a backup system for the relatives, not only the patient, is the key that makes a home care program successful.

Also necessary is a backup system for those of us who are doing the home care. There is a "domino theory" in a positive and negative sense for caregivers, as well as for patients and families.

If those of us who are doing home care receive support, too; if, for example, we are not simply convenience offshoots of the institution or hospital but are an integral part of it—serving on its planning committees, holding equally important committee chairmanships, and so forth, at *every* administrative level as well as at every clinical level—then the hospital can serve as a crucial resource for the home care team. Thus, mutually integrated, we can do much more for our patients. If the hospital system is to be trusted, it must be willing to reach out into the community with all of its relevant resources, giving care to the patient at home and yet remaining available always—ready not only to avert the feelings of abandonment that can threaten a terminal patient but also to *guarantee* the bed and room at such a time when, and if, they may become necessary. The ideal is, perhaps, a system that offers the possibility of a compromise—home care for as long as it is feasible and for as long as it can provide the greatest emotional and physical support for the patient and family—and then, if it must be so, or would be better so, a familiar caregiving hospital team committed to preserving a sense of "caring" continuity within the hospital and ever present there.

⚮⚮⚮ Preface

Twentieth-century advances in medical research, information, and technology have served to elevate the importance of hospital care for the acutely and chronically ill patient, but the result has been dependence on the hospital as a place where recovery may be assured and where terminal care should be given. This volume describes viable alternatives to the traditional in-hospital programs for terminal care, among them home care programs and also hospice-type programs similar to those already operative in other parts of the world. The basic premise of the contributing authors is that terminal care can be provided in effective and humanitarian ways beyond the walls of an institution and that professional caregivers can provide a variety of options for a higher degree of emotional and physical support for patients and their families when death approaches.

Some hospitals, with vision and a sensitivity to patient-care needs, assumed leadership roles in establishing active home care programs in the 1940s. In the next 20 years, programs by the American Cancer Society in various cities in the United States and Cancer Care, Inc., in New York City, were inaugurated. However, the inability of our society to come to terms with its own feelings about death and the dying and to develop a perspective on life and the living were reflected, to some extent, in an actual fear of giving care to the terminal patient at home. As presented in this book, the participation of homemaker associations, and social service and health service agencies has helped to allay some of these fears and alter negative attitudes.

Currently, there is a trend toward caring for the terminally ill at home. There is a growing interest in substantiating the validity of home care programs and in acknowledging the rights of dying patients and their family members to exercise a choice both in the type of care and in the place where it is to be given. In sharing their experiences, their knowledge and observations, the authors attest herein to the soundness and purposefulness of a system that facilitates continuity of care in familiar surroundings while avoiding the destructive effects of separation on family bonds which occurs when the patient remains in the hospital.

The Professional Standards Review Organization, now prominent in the establishment of health-care standards, has highlighted the gaps in a health-care system that fails to give due recognition to those resources required by the patient after the acute phase of illness is over. The continuing care needed by the terminally ill makes them the most vulnerable of all patients—vulnerable not only to personal indignities and dehumanization but also to most oppressive financial burdens. Providing care for them evokes anguish from the physician, the nurse, and the social worker largely because in too many areas there is a total lack of resources—either institutional or home-care oriented—to provide compassionate care for these patients and their families. There is little relevance in emphasizing cost containment in hospital care without exploring the positive aspects of a system that can be expanded outside the walls of the hospital.

When new modes of therapy seemed to promise cure and, in all too many situations, compromised the values of humane care when cure could not be achieved, death became a topic to be avoided and the dying became disenfranchised members of society. The impact upon our consciousness of attention addressed to psychosocial issues of terminal care during the past 10 years has made death and the dying process more acceptable as topics for discussion and investigation. As demonstrated by this book, home care involves many dimensions beyond the actual physical care given to the dying patient. Family members become involved in unaccustomed housekeeping roles when a mother is the patient; neighbors become involved, as providers of respite for those who must confront daily the imminence of a significant loss. The ultimate goals are an atmosphere of comfort and the maintenance of social participation within the home of a dying patient. Of particular importance is the support to be offered to spiritually strengthening interpersonal relationships—whether between parents and children, family members and friends, or husband and wife. Further, problems affecting the sexual activities of spouses who truly love each other when one suffers from the weakening onslaughts of a terminal disease are defined and solutions are proposed.

Above all, the substitution of home care for institutional care is offered as more than an unfulfilled promise. In addressing the concept and offering models for salutory home care, the authors of this book have demonstrated the best that is available today and have offered a base for future programs that can be supported by an informed public, enlightened legislation, and dedicated professionals.

The Editors

Home Care

Part I

Home Health Care

≋≋≋ 1

Home Health Care
and the Quality of Life

Leo Jivoff, Josephine A. Lockwood, Edith Oakes,

Mollie Schwartz, Janet Starr,

and Odessa Thompson

Modern in-home health care can make a critical and unique contribution to the quality of life of those whose lives are drawing to a close. This was the conclusion reached by a multidisciplinary committee of the Coalition for Home Health Services in New York State considering home health care and its impact on the quality of life of the dying patient. A nurse, a social worker, a home health aide, two physicians, and a home economist—all with long experience in home health care—agreed that most people who so wish may and should be maintained advantageously and comfortably at home as death approaches.

The fundamental requirement is a home setting that the patient alone defines as satisfactory. Like the determination of motivation,

Summary of Plan for Coalition for Home Health Services in New York State.

the patient's interpretation of the style, comforts, appearance, and accoutrements of home is the unarguable determinant of appropriateness. Equally fundamental in most, but not all, situations is the presence of an involved and cooperative family. To these bases can now be added a professional team to provide the medical and nursing treatment, psychosocial support, and ancillary services and to act as a source of responsibility for organizing the necessary personnel, equipment, and other resources needed to provide adequate coverage. There must, moreover, exist in the community the necessary services and the payment mechanisms to make them available to the patient. The resulting care can be tailored to the individual's particular needs and requirements. His sense of worth and independence will be encouraged with this increased opportunity to affirm life until its termination. The family will similarly benefit.

It is truer today than ever before that most persons who are nearing the end of life have lived long. Robert Butler (1975) attacks "the myth of serenity" regarding old age by pointing out that older persons experience more stress than any other age group and that these stresses are often devastating. Depression, anxiety, psychosomatic illness, paranoia, garrulousness, and irritability are frequent reactions to external stresses. Thus, there is a special need to attempt to reduce the feelings of loneliness and depression, to reinstate self-respect, revive old pleasures, reactivate social drives, reawaken intellectual interests, and redevelop some interest in community life.

Home health care helps to satisfy these needs, especially for the person admitted to a hospital or nursing home for care during an acute and postacute stage of illness. Confusion, disorientation, and withdrawal may occur swiftly in institutional settings. In some cases the expectations and demeanor of the professionals caring for the patient encourage passivity and dependence. In the institution a patient is ministered to by a variety of persons. Various time-effort studies have established that, in many hospitals and most nursing homes, the overwhelming proportion of personal bedside care is rendered by the least trained, least educated member of the nursing staff, the nurse's aide, who provides as much as 80 percent of the care. The licensed practical nurse may provide 15 percent, and the registered nurse, now spending most of her time with administrative and managerial duties, about 5 percent. The patient has little or no voice in what is done; usually he is told little and so does not understand. He is separated from his family and familiar surroundings. For the dying patient the special loneliness of the hospital is a cruel additional burden. Regulations limit visits by families and friends and eliminate children's visits. Doctors and nurses, unaccepting and embarrassed by death, struggling with the needs of the acutely ill, illogically concerned about the abuse of analgesics, magnify the isolation, and often the pain, of the dying patient. Although care at home may not be the universal solution, it is, despite shortcomings, better for most persons than care in an institution.

Home is truly a person's castle. There one is master. Within one's home, humble though it may be, one has the security of being surrounded by familiar objects—objects that have meaning and value to oneself alone. They stir memories. Only in one's own home does one have the freedom to eat what one desires when one desires it. Only here does one have the freedom to bathe, dress, and sleep when one wishes.

If the patient is a member of a family, he resumes his position within the family constellation after hospitalization, even though his role may be limited by disability and sometimes altered by his becoming the center of attention and concern. He has the opportunity to "set his house in order." Most people are aware of impending death whether told or not. Home care permits a period of shared grief. This period is particularly important for the family, since it tends to shorten the period of bereavement for them. The family members are also given the opportunity to avoid their own sense of guilt by contributing in some way, large or small, to the situation.

Where there is no family, extended family such as friends and neighbors will usually visit. They bring the outside world to the homebound. The patient, in turn, is tempted to look his best for these visitors; he is motivated to maintain his grooming. This, in turn, enhances his self-respect and tends to decrease feelings of depression. The homemaker-home health aide is often invaluable in such situations, since she offers continuity of contact as a person who is interested in this particular person as a human being. The patient no longer feels hopeless, abandoned, unwanted.

Home care, with the assistance of a home health aide, may permit a breadwinner family member to continue to work. Consequently, family stability on the economic level is maintained. The presence and services of the home health aide have frequently averted physical and emotional breakdown in the surviving family member.

Those observing home health care at first hand can cite striking examples of patients whose problems diminish or vanish when they are back in the security of their own homes. The diagnosis and prognosis do not change; the person's outlook does, because he becomes a person and a part of the family again.

Successful home health care for the person who will not recover requires, therefore, a home to go to where the patient will feel secure, a cooperative family, the availability of the needed home health services, and coordinated efforts and frequent communication by the home care team.

The home must exist, of course. There are almost no homes in which insurmountable physical barriers make care of the patient impossible. In most instances minor adjustments in the home or in the plans for care will make it suitable. Furniture may be rearranged to permit movement in a wheelchair or walker; a commode may be used where access to a bathroom is impossible. Handbars are easily installed.

Some equipment may be necessary and helpful, but care must be taken not to create an institution at home. This can happen when unnecessary equipment is used to relieve the feelings of insecurity on the part of family members. It can also happen when family members or others caring for the patient foster dependence by trying to do too much for him and by not permitting him to take part in decision making.

A most critical element in successful home health care is the willingness of the family to have the ill member at home and to participate in his care. A loving, dedicated family can be helped to overcome feelings of inadequacy or fear and can easily be trained to assume most of the patient care. Knowing what to expect, where they can turn for help in an emergency, and what the patient should be expected to do for himself will help them feel comfortable in providing care. Family members must be helped to assist where needed but helped also to guard against exhausting themselves physically and emotionally.

A word here about family willingness. As with many decisions made by families about posthospital care, attitudes of hospital-based physicians, nurses, social workers, and others may profoundly affect their choice. It is probably more true than not that hospital staffs subtly influence families to make institutional choices by themselves, deciding early in the course of hospital care that further institutional care is appropriate. In essence, they do not allow a choice to be made and provide a frightened family with a way out.

What about a hostile or indifferent family? Someone should try to work with such a family if the patient desires it and encourage participation to the best of their ability. Even token help, such as a regular telephone call, will help lighten the burden of guilt that may be felt later. Really hostile people should not, however, be inflicted on one another.

It is here that the home care team comes into play. The makeup of the team will be determined by the needs of the person being cared for and those of his family. Evaluation and regular reevaluation will result in changes in service delivery as indicated. The team will probably have as its key members a physician, a nurse, a social worker, and a home health aide. Therapists, clergy, the mobile laboratory technician, the friendly visitor, and many others may also help at one time or another. Coordination of the necessary services is usually assigned to the home health agency, which is then responsible for seeing that there is communication and understanding between all the caring and helping people. This communication should include the patient and family members, as well as home health personnel.

The physician is responsible for managing the care plan and for controlling pain. The rule about control of pain should be a simple one: any pain is unacceptable. Drugs must be provided in such dosage and frequency that the patient remains pain free. The physician should inform other team members what the patient knows of his diagnosis and of approaching death. The physician and family should decide whether the patient should be told. Whether he has been or not, the patient may know or suspect the truth. He may ask questions designed to probe or test. Such questions should be answered with honesty but, when necessary, with indirectness.

The social worker on the home care team and the nurse attempt to gain understanding of the patient and his family to arrive at an appropriate treatment plan. They are alert to the changing needs of the patient and his family and assist accordingly. They are highly supportive of the patient, the family, and the aide during this crucial period in the life of each member of the family. They help each express anger and frustration, fears and feelings of helplessness. The family is given emotional support so that it can remain intact.

The social worker does whatever she can to maintain family stability in this time of upheaval and impending loss. She may help the family locate sources of payment for the necessary services. She counsels family members and the patient as they deal with the stresses and changes resulting from the illness. The social worker will continue to work with the family after the death of the patient until an acceptable adjustment has been reached, if this help is needed. Too frequently this phase of treatment is overlooked and the case is closed abruptly when the patient dies. Studies have shown that the first year after the death of a close relative is a critical one. The incidence of emotional and physical breakdown and the mortality rate are higher for this group. Where indicated, treatment of the bereaved must, therefore, be continued.

The care given by the nurse on the home care team has many variables. Often the physician can be only at the other end of the phone and must depend on her observation and judgment. With him, she shares the responsibility for comfort, freedom from anxiety and pain, and perhaps the final decision to stay at home or be hospitalized. Many physicians know the patient and family from an office visit, clinic visit, or hospitalization. They may not know the resources of the home, the family, or extended family and so may depend on the nurse or other team members for this information. When the family is able and wants to give care, the nurse must recognize this and give only those directions that are needed for patient comfort, at the same time not allowing family members to overestimate their physical and emotional strengths. Intervention by the nurse, with an aide assigned for personal care or household tasks, extends the time for "caring" for both patient and family.

Though the nurse may not give the nursing care, the laying on of hands, that many expect, she does carry out the skilled services of her profession. Included in these skills, as well as nursing procedures, are the respect for other's rights, for their own beliefs, lifestyles, and cultural differences. A nurse skilled in communication is a good listener, is aware of what patient and family know, what they wish to talk about and when. Following these leads, she gives or arranges for changing care, knowing full well that, though she cannot always make the patient more comfortable physically or emotionally, there is much comfort in the presence of a concerned person.

The home health aide, a trained paraprofessional, is the team member who has most frequent and prolonged contact with the patient and his family. She performs personal care and homemaker tasks under supervision. She shares her observations regarding changes in physical condition and changes in attitude and behavior of the patient and the family with the members of the team who visit the home. She attempts to establish a calm yet cheerful atmosphere within the home. She may be the one who keeps the house running. She usually develops a close relationship with the patient. She shows that she cares. The aide must, however, guard against becoming emotionally involved or assuming the prerogatives of a family member. The home health aide often spends time listening to the patient as he relives his life or expresses his feelings. Most aides who work well with dying patients are mature, giving, compassionate women or men who have coped successfully with changes in their own lives. Some have a missionary feeling and a strong religious motivation.

The responsibilities outlined here for various team members are not rigidly assigned. Many home health programs lack the resources to offer a spectrum of professional services. Many patients may not need the services of all team members. Professional involvement in some instances may need to be limited to consultation with the nurse, aide, or other team member. A nurse may assume some of the functions of the social worker when there is not one on the staff.

Such stopgap measures should be recognized as such. The goal should be a multidisciplinary team effort if home health care's unique potential is to be realized.

A team effort draws on the different perspective, approach, background, and training of each of the team members. Each has something different to contribute, but the differences blur as they work together. A team effort not only gives the patient the benefit of care by persons trained in specific disciplines but also results in a total approach to him by any one of the team members. As the team process works, the effect of each member upon the others becomes apparent. The nurse and social worker begin to observe and absorb each other's knowledge and perspective, for example. Soon someone listening to a team conference would find it difficult to identify the disciplines of its members. Each team member sees the patient as an individual and recognizes a wider variety of his needs and the kinds of help required to satisfy them.

A strength of home health care is that the amount and kind of care given can be tailored to the individual, changing as his condition changes, while his home remains the site of care to the very end.

The Coalition was organized to spur development of the necessary range of services and payment sources so that individualized care could be available to all those for whom care at home was the treatment of choice. The Coalition has brought together more than 100 organizations in support of this effort. It has identified the health care services, the specialized health services, and the general services that should be available in our communities so that the services a patient needs may be brought together and he may be cared for at home. The Coalition has worked, and continues to work, for more nearly adequate financing of home health care and for inclusion of home care as an integral part of the continuum of health care.

The statement of philosophy adopted by the Coalition says, in part:

– that a person's home be viewed as an appropriate setting for the provision of health care services and that, when care at home is not appropriate, quality institutional care be available;
– that in-home care be an integral part of the community health care system,

with adequate provision for entry into the system and with provisions for ease of movement to and from any element within the system;
– that preventive, supportive, and treatment services be included in the range of in-home services made available and accessible to those with health-related problems;
– that the services provided be centralized and coordinated for the benefit of the individual and with the involvement of the family and the appropriate disciplines;
– that the sources of financing and coverage for in-home services be increased to remove all financial and other barriers;
– that human values be given priority, although the cost-effectiveness of home health services must not be ignored;
– that in-home services be provided in circumstances that are safe and effective.

To ensure that the individual remains the focus of in-home services, it is essential that

– the needs of the individual determine that services to be provided to him in his home and that
– the individual, family members, and professions participate jointly in making decisions about the place, type, and extent of care and services needed and received.

These principles are generic ones, applicable to all those requiring in-home care. They will help to safeguard the quality of life to its end.

Reference

Butler, R. 1975. *Why Survive?* New York: Harper & Row.

🐿🐿🐿 2

A Historical Perspective
on Home Health Care

Earland Cyrus

It is indeed appropriate at this time to consider the fact of death in a society that would deny the existence of a power outside of itself and would reinforce that denial by minimizing the effect that death has on those who survive. Thus the concept of thanatology—the process of dying and its effect on the patient and survivors—is of significance to those engaged in rendering health services at home.

Home care is the rebirth of an ancient and honorable concern on the part of the family (in a limited individual sense and also the family in the larger sense of the human society) toward one of its members who is passing through a period of illness. The hoped for end is restoration to maximum activities of daily living commensurate with the patient's age. However, because the age of most patients who make up the home care population is in the sixth decade or over, death is usually the end result of the care activity.

In my experience in home care, we endeavor to teach our patients to live with their disability and to cope with the loss of function, but we fail to prepare them for the final loss. In an earlier generation, when one could not boast of a technology that seemed to stay the hands of death, those who took care of the dying sick were not reluctant to talk of the dying process and make preparations for it, that is, location and site of burial, clothing, role of each member of the family, and so on.

Our modern society, which, in general, has scoffed at the concept of life after death has left itself without a hope upon which the dying can lean or with which the living can rationalize its loss. Most ancient societies were aware of this hope. The ancient Babylonians and Egyptians provided for the afterlife, as demonstrated in their funeral customs. The Patriarch Job cried out, "If a man dies shall he live again?" (Job 11) and then triumphantly answered the question by declaring, "I know my redeemer liveth. . . ."

It has been determined by research that two thoughts weigh on the mind of the dying: the fear of loneliness, of being abandoned, and prolonged pain. The second is more tolerable than the first.

As a corollary to the fear of abandonment is the grief associated with the loss of persons in the family structure. Grief after loss is a typical human phenomenon; the child who loses a favorite toy or other cherished object exhibits this reaction to some degree.

There is a special role to be assumed by the home care organization in this new appraisal of death and its effects. Home care is not new. In the nineteenth century most care of the sick was done in the home environment. Since folk medicine was the vogue rather than the exception, the mother or oldest female assumed the role of nurse and doctor up to the point where, owing to the severity or duration of the illness, professional care by a doctor was sought. Of course, in those days the profession did not have very much more to offer. Other members of the family, friends, and neighbors supplied the social and fiscal support to the dying person.

At that time the hospital or asylum was considered the place of last resort where only the homeless and derelict were taken care of. In the latter part of the century the wealthy and more sophisticated elements of society began to drop attendance on the sick at home, even though they could afford to hire attendants and request the doctor's presence at will. This trend was fostered by the fact that having the sick dying at home restricted social activities; moreover, the medical profession began to improve its knowledge of life processes, and the inappropriateness of certain care in the home stimulated the construction of institutions for care (which the wealthy supported). It was not long before the lower economic groups began to demand an upgrading of the almshouse or asylum to render better care so that the poor, too, could be hospitalized. Thus, we entered the twentieth century with a hospital- or institution-oriented society.

The resurgence of care at home, especially for those who have had a period of hospital care, has been generated by economic factors rather than humanitarian ones. It was conceived to be a cheaper mode of caring for the patient who no longer depended on the sophisticated equipment and services of an institution, and it freed bed space for acutely ill patients.

The typical home care agency now provides the following services: (1) physician care and supervision, (2) intermittent skilled nursing care, and (3) social service—economic care. These three services are basic. In addition there are (4) physiotherapy, (5) housekeeping, and (6) personal care. We see here a revival of those services rendered by family, friends, and neighbors in more primitive societies.

In our urban society and especially in the so-called ghetto or inner city most of those persons being serviced by a home health services agency are the sick aged. To this group of persons bereavement is not foreign; many have lost members of their family and close friends. They have adjusted to some degree and now are awaiting their own demise. Many of them grasp at the people who are servicing them as filling a void, either as a member of the family or trusted friend; this is especially true with those patients who have spent a year or more under care, while the process of death slowly evolves.

This compensation for bereavement by the patient and family, if any, points up the need for the agency to be ethnically oriented to enter somewhat into the patterns of mourning of various groups of people. For example, the agency in Harlem (New York City) deals with a group of blacks, but within this group is a diversity of backgrounds, namely, Southern United States, Caribbean, Hispanic. To each of these divisions the dying person is seen in a different perspective as related to himself, to the family, friends, and neighbors. The

religious milieu is also a factor in this process of relating to the
dying.

Another element in home care is the role of the family in caring
for the dying or terminal patient. Again we must reiterate the fact, although almost a cliché, that the modern family has very little of the
cohesiveness that marked the family of a century ago. The habitation
of grandparents, parents, and children in a single environment has
disappeared. Those persons in the home care program who have
children or nephews or nieces living with them are not much better
off, because the younger members have their own welfare at stake.
As a result the home care team often has to lend support to these persons to encourage their participation in the care of the dying patient.

Every death entails some change in the status of the surviving
kin, the relationship of the dying person being an important factor;
that is, is it a mother, father, sister, brother, or aunt? The team must
be aware of what the death means to the members of the family involved. Will a burden be lifted, spelling freedom? Will there be guilt
for not having done enough? Can the team offer a means of catharsis?
Is there a change in the pattern of behavior on the part of all parties
involved? These are all questions that the home care team will have
to be knowledgeable about if it hopes to make a contribution to society in this area.

Death, with its grief, shame, and guilt, has corresponding elements of anger and rage. These emotions are often repressed and can
prolong the period of grief. Thus, we see the bereaved person both
blaming himself for the demise and being angry for being left alone.

How do we cope with dying and the fear of death? As hinted
earlier, the old custom of permitting the patient to die at home enabled the person to be surrounded by concerned folk, with life's taking place in a familiar and beloved environment. In this setting less
adjustment is required for the dying person. The members of the family can continue to communicate their concern and hopes by physical
and verbal contact. The home care team must learn to appreciate
what the home environment means and not undertake to make radical
changes in the context of making the patient more comfortable.
Members of the family must be cultivated to learn their reactions,

strengths, and weaknesses in order to guide and use these qualities for the benefit of the patient. The team must also be aware of the need of the patient to talk and volunteer his own philosophy of life and death and must be conscious of the mood of the person from hour to hour and day to day.

There is a growing consensus that the dying and those concerned with their care at home, whether family or professional home care team, are subject to psychological stress that must be dealt with or ventilated, if they are to avoid psychological or physical suffering or both. At present, death and mourning are still viewed with reluctance by many. Showing emotional responses is felt to be out of character in a dynamic society. However, individual reports by team members would negate this idea. The gratitude that patients and their family express at being able to talk to someone about their fears and grief is often overwhelming.

Finally, the process of dying should be considered as a part of living and not as a traumatic end. Grief and gratification should be recognized as intrinsic parts of the process. Those who must deal with the dying on a professional level—the home care team—must be trained or at least exposed to the ethical issues involved and the behavior patterns of grief and bereavement.

ᔍᔍᔍ 3

Dying Is a Family Affair

Jeanne Quint Benoliel

Many individuals and families in today's technically oriented world are not well prepared for the stresses and strains introduced by a life-threatening illness. Perhaps the majority have had limited opportunity to learn how to handle themselves in the face of death and dying in great measure because the dying are so effectively segregated from the living. The exceptions are, of course, the underprivileged peoples in the Third World countries, where living and dying exist side by side. Rather in contrast, people in Western societies not only have little direct experience with dying but also are socialized to view human death as a phenomenon to be controlled by machines and active interventions. In the United States in particular the worship of lifesaving activity has led to a proliferation of life-prolonging procedures and the involvement of a great many professionals and laypeople in the almost unrestrained use of cardiopulmonary resuscitative techniques.

Indeed, people today are socialized into a way of life that places

Prepared for presentation as the third Alexander Ming Fisher lecture held at the College of Physicians and Surgeons of Columbia University, New York, New York, on April 21, 1976. Reference is made to research supported by grant awards M-5495 from the National Institute of Mental Health and NU00024 from the Division of Nursing, DHEW.

a high value on lifesaving actions, death control procedures, and simultaneously the importance of self-control in the face of strong and conflicting emotions. As Ariès (1974) points out, people in the twentieth century are ill prepared for the suffering and concrete problems that the crisis of dying brings into being. The shock of coping with the major changes in roles and role relationships produced by the terminal stage of illness is compounded by a lack of knowing how to behave comfortably with the person who is facing death.

Given the death-denying and death-controlling nature of American society in the 1970s, the general tendency to depersonalize human death and dying is not very surprising. The result for the person facing death can be social isolation or confinement to an institution or transfer to an intensive care setting without necessarily much choice in the decision (Benoliel, 1974). In a word the outcomes for the dying person are not very pleasant, but families too find themselves caught in a situation marked by tension and strain. The introduction of a life-threatening situation exerts tremendous pressure on a family's existing social system of supporting relationships and can easily lead to a disruption of personal and familial goals (Cancer Care, Inc., 1973).

My interest in the adaptations required of individuals and families in response to sudden death and life-threatening illness began some 20 years ago when a sudden and unexpected death brought havoc into my own family and initiated many personal reflections about the finiteness of human existence—especially my own. Since then, I have been fortunate in having had many opportunities to broaden my understanding of the complex nature of human responses to adversity and change. These understandings have emerged out of social research designed for understanding the personal and social meanings of life-threatening illness to the various persons involved in a given situation, contacts with students during their struggles to come to terms with their thoughts and feelings about death and dying, and my work as a clinical practitioner with patients and families living under the special pressures imposed by advanced malignant disease.

Out of these experiences I have come to appreciate the problems that people face in remaining human with one another when confronted with a death-related crisis. I have also come to respect the human capacity to cope with difficult transitions in positive rather than negative ways when help and guidance are made available to the major participants. As Strauss (1975) has observed, progressive illnesses create multiple problems of daily living and often necessitate major changes in life-styles and family living patterns. It is not the strictly medical aspects of the illness that cause the families' problems. Rather it is the impingement of the disease/treatment on their interactions with each other, on their social and financial resources, on their normal activities and habits, and on their usual roles and role relationships. Coping with transition takes command of their lives and assumes a special urgency whenever individuals find themselves faced with a life-threatening crisis.

Death-Related Transitions

I examine three types of death-related transition, each of which impinges heavily on a family's established system of social relationships and store of fiscal and psychosocial resources. The three situations can be defined in these ways: (1) the impact and aftermath of sudden death, (2) the influence of unspoken death fears on family relationships, and (3) the interrelated effects of prolonged dying and social dependency. My purpose in discussing these three situations is to identify and describe the characteristics of the psychosocial crisis peculiar to each transition and the kinds of services that are needed by individuals and families to assist them in adapting to the social demands and personal changes imposed by these transitions.

I am focusing attention on the *needs for care* experienced by families in these situations as distinct from their needs for curative medical services and life-saving activity (Benoliel, 1976). That is, my comments are directed toward clarifying the impact of these death-related crises on completion of unfinished business, resolution or nonresolution of old conflicts, and other changes associated with preparation for the coming death or resolution of reactions to a death already completed.

As discussed on previous occasions (Benoliel, 1972), the present health care system in the United States is much better organized to implement the cure goals of practice than it is to offer person-centered care. By this I mean that the system is organized mainly for the diagnosis and treatment of disease, for the management of the person as an objective case, and for the implementation of medical treatments and related procedures *done to* people rather than with them. In general, the system is poorly organized to provide health care consumers with regular help geared to the subjective meanings of the disease experience, the welfare and well-being of the persons involved, and the delivery of activities designed and implemented *in collaboration with* the consumers.

As part of this commentary, I examine the concept of transition services as one approach for the creation of health care services designed to foster the delivery of person-centered services. I also explore the unique position held by nurses in the health care system and the value of nursing contributions to the achievement of care for many individuals and families who are living through the complex set of transitions known as dying, death, and bereavement.

The Impact and Aftermath of Sudden Death

The first of the transitions, sudden death, produces a major crisis for a family's system of social relationships precisely because it is unexpected. Because in this instance death (a major change) occurs without warning, all of the survivors suffer from a lack of opportunity to prepare for the change. Not uncommonly, many are left with the added psychological problem of unfinished business with the person who died. In addition the sudden death of a key member in a family social structure may initiate an immediate need for shifts in roles to keep the ongoing business of the family in operation. Let me illustrate these points by reference to my sister's death.

My sister, some four years younger than I, was in the eighth month of pregnancy with her fourth child. (The other three children were three, five, and seven years of age.) On a Sunday evening she complained to her husband of a very bad headache and went to the bedroom to rest for a while. Suddenly she cried out in agony, and he rushed to the bedroom to find her having a convulsion. With the help of a neighbor she was taken immediately to the emergency room of a nearby hospital for treatment. While still in the emergency room, she went into respiratory arrest and was rapidly put onto a life support system. Soon therafter she was taken to the operating room, where a caesarean section was performed, and, subsequently, a craniotomy was done to relieve what appeared to be a cerebral hemorrhage.

At the time of my arrival on Monday at noon, I found my brother-in-law clearly in a state of major upset. My sister was unconscious and breathing only with the assistance of a continuous respirator. The physician in charge indicated that she was unable to breathe on her own owing to a massive hemorrhage into the brain stem, and together we decided to discontinue the machine. Afterward my brother-in-law, his best friend and I sat for eight hours, waiting for her heart to stop beating. To emphasize the poignancy of this story, her dying took place on the obstetrical unit of the hospital in a room directly across from the nursery where her new baby had been sent.

This personal situation is used because it illustrates the special and stressful problems created for family systems when a key member of that system—the young mother in this case—is unexpectedly and permanently removed by sudden death. The husband not only has to deal with his personal reactions to the loss of an important relationship but also is confronted with the very difficult problem of what to do with four children under seven years of age. During the immediate postdeath period I stayed with him and the children, and considerable assistance was made available by the neighbors. Much more problematic was the need to find housekeeping and child care services on a long-term basis within the limitations of his income. The family social system experienced considerable disruption and strain during the postdeath year precisely because of the difficulties in finding child care services and in keeping the children together.

This personal experience can also point to the special problems that young children face after the death of a parent. In retrospect I am aware that the adults were all so caught up in their own reactions of shock and distress that they were unable to be very supporting to the children. That my sister's death had a profound effect on these youngsters was demonstrated in the regressive patterns of behavior shown by the three older children as they struggled to adapt to a style of living without their mother. Their father was caught in the difficult position of trying to be both mother and father and at the same time to find some kind of resolution for himself. My parents were psychologically shattered by the shock of this unexpected loss of their youngest child, and part of how they came to terms with the loss was to take the new baby into their home for a year.

The usefulness of this example is that it points to the heavy stress of unanticipated death during the productive years. Yet it is also clear that sudden death at any time poses great psychological and social problems for the survivors left behind. Responding to the loss of a husband who dies from a sudden heart attack can be difficult at any age; when that sudden death occurs through accidental injury or suicide or homicide, the psychosocial problems are compounded and intensified—especially when the survivors are left with many remnants of unfinished business such as that resulting from a quarrel or painful disagreement. The psychological aftermath of sudden death can also be intensified when the death takes place as part of a total and catastrophic disaster. As Lifton and Olson (1976) have described, the people who survived the massive destruction of the Buffalo Creek flood that destroyed an entire community were left with psychological patterns characterized by a pervasive sense of despair. When sudden death of a significant person occurs as part of a larger catastrophic event, the survivors have an added problem of dealing with strong feelings of guilt because they have survived.

When we consider the kinds of services needed by families for coping with this kind of tragic experience, it seems reasonably clear that the surviving persons all have need for support to enable them to deal with the psychological impact of sudden loss and major change on their self-perceptions and future orientations. Parkes (1971) has stated that what happens during the crisis stage of a major psychosocial transition strongly affects the subsequent course of an individual's life, including his relationships with other people. The definition of *support* used here comes from Robert S. Weiss (1976) and refers to the communication, verbal and nonverbal, extended by a helping person's indicating that the helper's background, knowledge, special expertise, experience, and understanding are available to the distressed individual as he or she struggles to come to terms with a personally disorganizing transitional crisis.

One reason, in my opinion, that many people have difficulty in achieving resolution of the loss of a significant person by means of sudden death is the nonavailability of support beyond the period immediately following the death. In other words, supporting people may be readily available during the period of immediate impact, but after the funeral the survivors are likely to find themselves pretty much on their own. According to my observations and personal experiences, people undergoing the psychosocial transition initiated by unexpected death are badly in need of personally supporting relationships for a prolonged period of time. In addition to psychological support per se, these people are often helped in their adjustments to this change by being given a realistic appraisal of the actual cause of death and the circumstances surrounding it. The valuable contribution made by public health nurses to the welfare and well-being of families following the loss of a baby through sudden infant death syndrome has been documented in the literature (Bergman, 1972).

My sister's death also illustrates well the broad range of assistance needed by young families in particular when the sudden death of a key person leaves a major gap in their set of roles and role relationships. Often these families need help in locating multiple resources to assist them in reorganizing their lives; the resources they need may include money, jobs, transportation, housekeeping services, and many others. The services they need are more than what are available in our traditional systems for the delivery of health care services. Furthermore, the services need to be readily available if they are to be of maximum assistance at the time of maximum need.

Family systems differ in their abilities to cope constructively with the stresses and strains imposed by unanticipated death. In studying the aftermath of these tragic events for families, Vollman and her associates (1971) found that those families able to use crisis intervention activities were atomized, nuclear families accustomed to the idea of professional help and having financial resources enabling them to use this assistance. A second group of families were observed to have a cohesive system of social supports coming from within the established subcultural group of which they were a part. In contrast, a third group of families—those with few social ties to the community—were resistant to crisis intervention and highly vulnerable to physical and social disorganization in response to the crisis posed by sudden death. These differences in adaptive capacities suggest that any plan for organized transition services should take account of differences in the coping abilities of various types of family social systems and probably should pay special heed to the needs for assistance of highly vulnerable groups and individuals such as those caught in the aftermath of major catastrophes or multiple losses (Benoliel, 1971).

Unspoken Death Fears and Family Relationships

A second critical type of death-related transition is a mode of adaptation to living with life-threatening illness characterized mainly by avoidance of open conversation about the underlying threat of death. Often this pattern of responding to forthcoming death takes the form of family members' deciding that the person with fatal illness is not to be given a full and true account of his diagnosis and prognosis. The common rationale for making this choice is protection of the person whose life is moving toward a close. Actually, it seems to me, this action does precisely the opposite by placing the individual in a situation in which fantasies and fears about death and the future replace knowledge about the reality of the situation. Indeed the decision by others to avoid open talk about the forthcoming death really protects them from having to deal directly with the personal concerns of the person who is dying. This choice for nondisclosure can also rather effectively keep them at a distance from their own deep feelings and concerns about the forthcoming death.

The outcomes of nondisclosure for the person who bears the fatal illness are social isolation and denial of opportunity for talking openly about the meaning of living and dying. Such a decision by family members and health care providers can effectively serve as an obstacle blocking the individual's opportunities to bring closure to his life according to his own set of wishes. Indeed when open discussion about the realities of death is constrained and hidden, the setting in which death takes place and the circumstances surrounding the final event are then determined by the choices and decisions of the other people who comprise the dying person's primary social relationships. Yet despite the best of intentions, these choices and decisions may or may not take account of the dying person's wishes, and sometimes they lead to stressful experiences not easily forgotten. For example, the inability of the parents of a young woman with advanced cystic fibrosis to face the reality of her progressive illness led to poor medical followup and eventually to a terrifying experience of her dying in a context of intensive lifesaving activity removed from those persons most important in her life (Benoliel, 1974).

Just as sudden death leads to shifts in roles and role relationships within a family, so also can the demands imposed by progressive fatal disease contribute to major changes in a family structure. As Anthony (1970) observed, a change of this nature can sometimes stimulate the creation of an interpersonal matrix marked by disorder and distrust. Unresolved and unspoken tensions and fears related to death directly influence the patterning of social relationships within a family, but sometimes these choices are not made at the conscious level. Rather, one can think of them as direct reflections of a basic death-denying theme in American society manifest in socializing practices that cause people to grow into adulthood quite unaware of their well-established behaviors of death avoidance. Studying one family in which the father's precarious health was such that he lived continuously on the brink of sudden death, Bermann (1973) found that the unspoken death fears experienced by the adults led to scapegoating as the family's way of coping with stress. The unfortunate result of this mode of adaptation was the disruptive influence it had on the personal and social development of the son who happened to be the scapegoating target. This example is important because it points to the high vulnerability of children to interpersonal exploitation in the context of forthcoming death. That is, when the adults in a family are unable to deal constructively with their death-related tensions and fear, children in that situation are liable to be caught in the crossfire of those stresses. For those who are concerned about the importance of preventive health services, the future lives of children enmeshed in the intricate webs of these high-stress family situations may well depend on whether something can be done to break through and alter communication patterns of scapegoating and other nonpositive approaches to family relationships.

Ideally perhaps, open communication about the reality of forthcoming death is a goal to be achieved, and yet many situations are not easily solved by simply advocating open awareness. For example, the problems of communication about the life-threatening aspects of illness can be very difficult when more than one person in the household is diagnosed in this direction, as can happen in families that have more than one child with cystic fibrosis. In one such family the parents found themselves living with the difficult problem of having one diagnosed child who looked and behaved remarkably well and another who was sickly in appearance and clearly moving rapidly toward the end of life. Like many parents in such a situation, these two did not talk openly with the children about the fatal nature of the illness. But it was equally clear that all of the family lived in an atmosphere of continuous tension associated with the underlying theme of forthcoming death.

As is often true in such situations, the mother's time was essentially committed to implementing the complex treatment regimen for the sickest boy, the father serving as backup support for her. The heavy treatment regimen required for cystic fibrosis in combination with the young boy's sickly appearance had affected the entire family, and sometimes the mother felt that the other children had lost out on certain activities because of it. She also commented that the other children were very good about living with the problem, and the family as a whole tried not to make a big deal out of it. This family had available to them an extensive social network of parents and other relatives providing thereby a readily available system of supporting relationships similar to those described by Caplan (1974). Although there was relatively little open conversation about impending death, the members were clearly aware of its reality, and they had modified their lives to accommodate its continuing demands.

Only when the boy became morose and withdrawn and refused to participate in his treatments did the mother find herself unable to function very well. Caught in the ambivalent feelings of wanting him to live and wanting him to die, she told the doctor she could not take the situation any more because the boy never smiled. When it became apparent that his dying would be prolonged, the doctor and parents together made a decision to remove him to the hospital "for the sake of the other children." Even to the end, these parents were unable to talk directly with the dying boy about his future; despite the availability of an extensive system of socially supporting relationships, they were not observed to alter their established pattern of nondisclosure. Such a shift, in my opinion, would depend on the opportunity to grapple with a complexity of strong and conflicting emotions in a supporting environment and to learn new ways of communicating with other people. Before we consider some approaches that have been found effective for helping dying people and their families to experiment with new patterns of communication, some additional observations about the interrelated effects of prolonged dying and progressive social dependency would appear to be useful.

Prolonged Dying and Progressive Social Dependency

Cancer is perhaps the prototype of death-related disease since so many people appear to equate dying with the experience of having cancer. As I learned in studying the processes whereby women adjust to a mastectomy during the first year after the surgery, the diagnosis for them meant learning to live with an uncertain future and with a nagging underlying concern about whether and when the cancer would return (Quint, 1963; Quint, 1964). As one of these women commented during her final interview:

You feel a tremendous weight hanging over you. I feel it, but not constantly. I have periods of—well, how can I say it intelligently? I'm hardly ever without the awareness of, the possibility of—even though I say no. But I don't dwell on it—though I do find that I'm very nervous which is not like my normal self. And I'm sure that a good bit of it goes to this problem.

From the personal perspective of the diagnosed person, cancer can be conceived as catastrophic because it produces major changes in living for him and his family. Dying begins for him when the diagnosis is bestowed. Often, however, the full impact of life-threatening disease is most acutely felt when personal and social changes imposed by the illness and treatment create the need for restructuring an established style of living to accommodate these needs for change. Fagerhaugh (1975) has shown how progressive emphysema contributes to a diminishing of energy resources associated with decreased breathing capacity and a progressive restriction of the person's ability to move about easily and to maintain active social involvement with other people. Writing about the impingements of chronic diseases in general, Strauss (1975, pp. 7–8) identified seven areas that created problems in daily living: (1) the prevention of medical crises and their management, (2) the control of symptoms, (3) the carrying out of prescribed treatment regimens without creating additional problems, (4) the prevention of social isolation or adaptation to it, (5) the adjustment to changes in the course of disease as takes place in response to exacerbations and remissions, (6) the efforts at normalizing interactions with other people, and (7) the problem of adequate funds to pay for treatment and make up for losses of income associated with having the illness.

In a sense, chronic illness of any type initiates a process of prolonged dying, though much of the time we do not define these illnesses in this way. As a psychosocial transition, progressive chronic disease is characterized by physical and physiological changes that over time reach a stage of such severity that the person bearing the disease finds himself in a state of enforced physical and social dependency. In advanced malignant disease the diagnosed person finds himself progressively depending on other people for help with a great many activities that previously he did for himself. The inability to provide self-care with intimate activities can be a blow to personal self-esteem, and yet this experience is commonplace for persons in the advanced stages of illness.

Pain and discomfort associated with progressive disease are often problems in need of solution, and once again the person with the cancer finds himself having to depend on other people to achieve relief. A common problem described by people with advanced cancer is social isolation—a sense of being cut off from talking about those things that really matter (McCorkle, 1973). Ironically, social isolation effectively cuts the person off from sharing his deep concerns and fears with other people, but it also cuts him off from conversations about ordinary, everyday kinds of things as well. Yet Feder (1965) makes the point that both kinds of social opportunities are important for maintaining hope as a human being.

The cancer patient is a victim of the people who surround him. The extent to which he finds help in coming to terms with his forthcoming death and in achieving the personal goals he has set for himself is greatly influenced by the choices and decisions of those persons who make up his important relationships. Yet the members of the family are also under the stresses imposed by the multiple and difficult problems introduced by progressive illness. Hoffman and Futterman (1971) have cogently detailed the conflicting pulls and difficult developmental tasks that families and patients face continually throughout the period of living with a fatal illness. Just as the person whose life is drawing to a close has special concerns and goals, so also do the persons to whom he or she has a significant relationship. Children and adolescents are highly vulnerable to the loss of a significant relationship, and yet children's needs for active participation in the dying transition commonly go unmet because the adults believe they are protecting them (Karon and Vernick, 1968; Share, 1972) or are too busy taking care of their own unmet needs (Benoliel, 1974).

May (1974) observed that the crisis of death becomes problematic for the dying person and those closest to him precisely because the crisis interferes with the very basis of their relationship. The quiet, dependent husband who has created his life around the wishes and whims of a dominant, talkative wife finds himself in a new situation of having a wife now dependent and helpless. In an odd way he finds himself living with a stranger and homesick for their old, established rituals of relationship, which have now gone forever. The shock of coping with the major changes in roles and role relationships produced by terminal illness is compounded for many by a lack of preparation for knowing how to behave in the presence of someone who is dying.

The problem faced by many cancer patients and their families is finding helping services organized to assist them in implementing the medical goals of treatment and simultaneously finding resolution for their many personal wishes, concerns, and social difficulties encountered as part of the process of living and dying. Being able to die at home, for example, can happen only when someone is available to provide the personal services and assistance required for physical comfort and emotional support. In my experience, the opportunity for the dying person to die at home depends on a family willing to have it happen, but, equally important, having access to a socially supporting network of helping relationships to provide a backup system of resources and people.

Not long ago I served as counselor to a woman who was in the final stages of dying of malignant melanoma and who wanted to die at home. Perhaps my most important contribution to her was to serve as listener and guide to her husband over the final three months of her life as he struggled to grapple with the stresses and strains of that period and still remain in open communication with her.

This woman was fortunate in having access to a wide variety of fiscal and social supports sufficient to assist her in achieving a personalized dying. These supports included private nurses around the clock to provide physical care, management of pain, and regular contacts with her physician, as these were needed. She had a husband committed to her goal of dying at home. She had available an extensive network of relatives and friends who visited her regularly until she no longer had the energy for it and who were actively involved in helping out with the small everyday tasks of living that so often are lost during the transition of dying. With progressive social dependency, for instance, a woman loses control over the management of her household, and being able to maintain some semblance of this control through directing other people can be an important part of the process of preparation for death. Most important of all, she had access to a corps of people willing to stay in open communication with her and wanting to help her in achieving a death on her own set of terms.

Transition Services and Nursing Contributions

Despite these examples of people able to achieve a personalized dying because of access to a family system committed to that goal, there are countless others whose experience is just the opposite. Some are elderly people locked into an impersonal system of services and lacking a person willing to serve as advocate for them. Others are members of family systems unable to adapt to the extreme pressures imposed by dying because of a lack of one or more necessary resources. Families such as these are ill equipped to cope with the personal and interpersonal changes imposed by dying, and it is families such as these that need transition services.

Central to the conceptual framework for transition services is a belief that the person with cancer has a right to participate in the choices and decisions affecting the illness and treatment, as well as the circumstances surrounding his final days of living. Opportunities for such participation depend on health care providers committed to the provision of personalized services through activities designed to coordinate the goals of care and cure. In this concept the nurse occupies a position of central importance as the facilitator of personalized care. Personalized care, as used here, aims toward helping the dying person fulfill three opportunities not easily found in our society: (1) to know what is happening to and around him and to be able to talk about its reality with someone who will listen, (2) to participate in decisions affecting his final days, and (3) to experience the pain of feeling bad instead of having to hide these feelings as a means of protecting other people from their own pain.

The introduction of nurses as communication links and intermediaries between dying patients and families and the many other providers in the health care system is nothing new to nursing. From time immemorial, nurses have functioned in the social interface between consumers and their complex social networks outside the medical system and the physicians and other providers organized as a system of specialized services. The concept of transition services does make explicit the key functions performed by nurses in the delivery of person-centered services to dying patients and families as they move into a new energy-draining social experience with its unexpected and shifting demands. In a pragmatic sense the role projected for these nurses consists of a combination of public health, mental health, and physical assessment skills and an ability to accept responsibility for *continuity of care* through coordinating activities and resources and facilitating the flow of communication among the principal persons involved (Quint, 1965). That nurses can function in this capacity has been well described by Dancull (1973) out of her own experiences with terminal patients at home and by Donovan and Pierce (1976, pp. 25–43) with reference to persons dying of cancer.

A service of this nature should probably not be hospital based but would ideally be organized as an ambulatory service having interlocking ties to various hospitals, nursing homes, and other institutions providing care to dying people. Because nurses are accustomed to moving back and forth between patients' homes and formally organized health care settings, they have a combination of background and expertise essential for the creation of transition services. The delivery of support, instruction, coordinated activities, and care are accepted functions for nurses in general. These functions can assume a special significance when people need help in coping with the complex problems of prolonged dying and the dying patient's increased dependency on others around him (Ward, 1974; Benoliel, 1975).

The purposes of transition services might be stated as follows: (1) to increase the dying person's opportunities for goal achievement by making open communication easier among the various persons involved, (2) to improve the family's coping capacities by supplementing their social support system and/or guiding them in more effective use of the resources already available, (3) to assist the major participants in the dying to face and deal with the many strong feelings and conflicting demands they experience during the process, (4) to provide guidance in the management of physical changes associated with progressive illness and direction for the wise use of medications and medical treatments, (5) to communicate directly with various key providers so as to facilitate collaboration and coordination of the services being offered, and (6) to socialize the dying person and the members of his social network for the expected and unexpected elements of dying. The importance of nursing's contributions to the achievement of purposes such as these has not been well recognized by other health care professionals, nor are nurses always given credit for their perceptive balancing of the activities of care and cure. Yet these all-too-often hidden talents and capabilities can make the difference between a depersonalized experience of dying and the achievement of vigor in living until the very end. Transition services depend on nurses who have flexibility of approach and an ability to make rapid shifts in priorities to accommodate the changing needs of people living under circumstances of prolonged stress.

References

Anthony, E. J. 1970. "The Impact of Mental and Physical Illness on Family Life." *American Journal of Psychiatry* 127 (August):138–46.

Ariès, P. 1974. "Death Inside Out." *The Hasting Center Studies* 2 (May): 3–18.

Benoliel, J. Q. 1971. "Assessments of Loss and Grief." *Journal of Thanatology* 1 (May–June):182–94.

Benoliel, J. Q. 1972. "Nursing Care for the Terminal Patient: A Psychosocial Approach." In *Psychosocial Aspects of Terminal Care*, eds., B. Schoenberg et al., pp. 145–61. New York: Columbia University Press.

Benoliel, J. Q. 1974. "The Dying Patient and the Family." In *The Patient, Death, and the Family*, eds., S. B. Troup and W. A. Greene, pp. 111–23. New York: Scribners.

Benoliel, J. Q. 1975. "The Terminally Ill Child." In *Comprehensive Pediatric Nursing*, eds., G. Scipien et al., pp. 423–40. New York: McGraw-Hill.

Benoliel, J. Q. 1976. "Care, Cure and the Challenge of Choice." In *The Nurse as Caregiver for the Terminal Patient and His Family*, eds., A. Earle et al., pp. 9–30. New York: Columbia University Press.

Bergman, A. B. 1972. "Sudden Infant Death." *Nursing Outlook* 20 (December):775.

Bermann, E. 1973. *Scapegoat: The Impact of Death-Fear on an American Family.* Ann Arbor: University of Michigan Press.

Cancer Care, Inc. 1973. *The Impact, Costs, and Consequences of Catastrophic Illness on Patients and Families.* New York: The National Cancer Foundation, Inc.

Caplan, G. 1974. *Support Systems and Community Mental Health.* New York: Behavioral Publications.

Dancull, M. V. 1973. "The Role of the Nurse in the Care of the Terminal Patient Through a Home Care Program." Unpublished master's thesis, The University of Maryland.

Donovan, M. I. and S. G. Pierce. 1976. *Cancer Care Nursing.* New York: Appleton-Century-Crofts.

Fagerhaugh, S. 1975. "Getting Around with Emphysema." In *Chronic Illness and the Quality of Life*, ed., A. L. Strauss, pp. 99–107. St. Louis: C. V. Mosby.

34   Jeanne Quint Benoliel

Feder, S. L. 1965. "Attitudes of Patients with Advanced Malignancy." New York: Group for the Advancement of Psychiatry. Symposium No. 11.

Hoffman, I. and E. U. Futterman. 1971. "Coping with Waiting: Psychiatric Intervention and Study in the Waiting Room of a Pediatric Oncology Clinic." *Comprehensive Psychiatry* 12 (January):67–81.

Karon, M. and J. Vernick. 1968. "An Approach to the Emotional Support of Fatally Ill Children." *Clinical Pediatrics* 7 (May):274–80.

Lifton, R. J. and E. Olson. 1976. "The Human Meaning of Total Disaster. The Buffalo Creek Experience." *Psychiatry* 39 (February):1–18.

McCorkle, R. 1973. "Coping with Physical Symptoms of Patients with Metastatic Breast Cancer." *American Journal of Nursing* 74 (June):1034–38.

May, W. 1974. "The Metaphysical Plight of the Family." *The Hastings Center Studies* 2 (May):19–30.

Parkes, C. M. 1971. "Psycho-social Transitions." *Social Science and Medicine* 5 :101–15.

Quint, J. C. 1963. "The Impact of Mastectomy." *American Journal of Nursing* 63 (November):88–91.

Quint, J. C. 1964. "Mastectomy: Symbol of Cure or Warning Sign?" *GP* 29 (March):119–24.

Quint, J. C. 1965. "Institutionalized Practices of Information Control." *Psychiatry* 28 (May):119–32.

Share, L. 1972. "Family Communication in the Crisis of a Child's Fatal Illness." *Omega* 3 (August):187–201.

Strauss, A. L. 1975. *Chronic Illness and the Quality of Life*. St. Louis: C. V. Mosby.

Vollman, R. et al. 1971. "The Reactions of Family Systems to Sudden and Unexpected Death." *Omega* 2(2):101–6.

Ward, A. W. M. 1974. "Terminal Care in Malignant Disease." *Social Science and Medicine* 8:413–20.

Weiss, R. S. 1976. "Transition States and Other Stressful Situations: Their Nature and Programs for Their Management." In *Support Systems and Mutual Help: Multidisciplinary Explorations,* eds., G. Caplan and M. Killilea. New York: Grune and Stratton, 1976.

Part II
The Needs of Patients and Families

༅༅༅ 4

Working with Dying Patients and Their Families

Josephine K. Craytor

Any discussion of working with the dying individual and his family that is relevant for the health professions must consider not only the dying person and the people most important to him but also the professional caregivers in order to improve the care provided. This chapter is concerned with ways in which health professionals can become more comfortable and probably more effective in working with dying patients and family members.

I should like to suggest some objectives for experiences aimed at improving care of the dying by helping us as caregivers continue to grow, including:

1. Show increased self-respect and confidence in our own common sense by setting limits to expectations of self, patient, and family.
2. Recognize the relevance to our personal goals of working with the dying person.
3. Foster the ability to change and grow, in ourselves and in others.
4. Increase our belief in the value of our own work.
5. Allow ourselves to feel concern for our own feelings, as well as those of the patient and family, during terminal illness and after death.

6. Increase confidence in our ability to stay with the dying person and involve ourselves appropriately in his care.

To achieve such objectives requires time, interpersonal interaction, and practice with patients and caring professional people. We can, in a short time, move only a bit closer to such objectives.

Let us look in more detail at the objectives outlined. First, to show increased self-respect and belief in our own common sense by recognizing our limitations and those of patient and family. Self-respect implies acceptance of feelings that may be far from noble. We may prefer not to be around sick patients or dying people, and we may fear becoming emotionally involved. If we can accept our own wish to avoid these things, it is easier to accept family behaviors and not to feel guilty about our feelings or angry toward the patient's family.

Once we can accept our behavior we can work on the second objective, recognizing the advantages to ourselves from assisting in the dying process. These may include increasing our sense of security in our ability to plan for and to handle threatening changes in ourselves, to handle our own fears, to get more satisfaction from working with patients in their imperfect efforts to deal with some of the problems, and to recognize that there is gratification in small successes in reaching toward a peaceful, positive acceptance.

If we can accept our limitations and those of others and recognize some of the positive returns that come to us in working with people, then we can move on to the third objective, developing our ability to change and grow. This may include becoming less afraid of feeling helpless and of recognizing our own vulnerability, our distaste for sickness and death, our reluctance to move toward people who are sick and dying, and our avoidance of anyone who feels rejected and bereft. Part of our avoidance is related to the fact that working with the dying person represents a threat to our occupational goals of curing and helping. If this is true, we have to look at the goals and decide whether helping people toward peace and comfort is a goal of equal importance. It is hard to accept the side effects of disease and treatment and to regard the loss of a patient as other than a defeat. We may be tempted to become involved in heroic lifesaving measures without assessing the real situation of the patient and the family.

Glaser and Strauss (1965) have noted that the dying trajectory or the perceived course of dying may differ from what is really going on. At present one of my neighbors is in the hospital. He has had a thoracotomy as the last of many diagnostic measures to determine the nature of a lung lesion. It was found that he has a large-cell carcinoma of the lung that is not operable because of its location. It is not a large lesion, and the plan has been made to treat him by radiation therapy. His wife believes, however, that he is dying, that she cannot take him home, and that she cannot do anything but wish that his course would be rapid and as painless as possible. She is even opposing the use of radiation therapy. She views his trajectory as a final, rapid decline, which is hardly the case, but she is proceeding as though it were real and is convincing him of this. At present it has not been possible to change her perception of what is going on or to show her how she might become involved. The husband is very depressed, and she is frightened. They have been surrounded by friends, but people are moving away, repelled by her rejection of him and by his depression. This can and will be changed, but it will take a great deal of effort.

The fourth objective is to develop a more positive attitude about one's own ability to be effective in, and to see the value of, our work with the dying patient and the family, as demonstrated by making a sincere effort to raise the level of care for the patient and the family members by using approaches that others have found successful. Some of the most effective learning comes directly from our patients, who can teach us about human strength and resourcefulness and often can support us. It may be useful to review some of the literature about the normal stages of grieving (Lindemann, 1944; Engel, 1964; Kübler-Ross, 1969) about what the threat of death means in terms of developmental tasks, about defense mechanisms that are useful to people in facing crises, and about the management of pain and other distressing symptoms. One demonstration of a positive attitude toward involvement with the dying patient is to meet with fellow professionals to discuss feelings, reactions toward dying patients, and problems in working with puzzling behavior of family and patients. It helps to share successes as well as problems, to reinforce feelings of competency and worth, and to note contributions that are made. As we become increasingly confident, we can tolerate higher levels of stress and be more effective as helpers.

Objective five is related to demonstrating a concern for the feelings of self, patient, and family during illness and after death. Sudnow (1967) found marked differences in the way in which dying patients were managed in a large county hospital and a smaller community hospital. He discussed social death as the state in which a person is abandoned, relegated to the dead while still physiologically alive. He saw many instances of this in a large, busy county hospital. Personnel might state concern but act in a way to demonstrate their feeling that the dying deserve no time.

One of the most effective ways to show concern for the dying patient's feelings is to listen, to assess his perception of what is happening, and to explore with him, as you both feel able, his real world, including his awareness of the deterioration in his physical status. It is tricky to empathize, to view the situation through the patient's eyes and not to identify with him to the extent that you feel things appear to him as they would to you in the same situation. I remember some years ago working with a 24-year-old woman who had a sarcoma of her maxillary sinus. She had had an antrectomy and drug therapy, and by the time she came to our medical center she had an unsightly tumor growing out of her right cheek and displacing her right eye upward, making her look quite hideous. I had known her over a period of many months during which she was amazingly courageous in dealing with her problems. She was ready to do anything that would slow the course of the disease. She was receiving some of the early chemotherapeutic drugs, with relatively little effect. She was hospitalized briefly at this time, and I went to see her. Several of the nurses met me as I came on the floor and one said, "We think Mrs. D. ought to be on suicide precautions." I was startled and asked them to tell me more about why they thought this. One young woman said, "Well, if I looked like that, I'd jump out the window." I tried to explain as gently as I could that, although Mrs. D. was difficult to look at, she was a remarkable and courageous woman and had been going to the greatest lengths to try and stay alive for the sake of her two-year-old daughter and her young husband. They continued to be uneasy, but as time went on they got beyond her grotesque appearance and found out what a wonderful woman she was.

Some of the familiar techniques are useful in helping, such as reflective counseling by which you repeat a word or phrase of the patient's as a question and let him elaborate on the idea as you listen without interpreting. This implies acceptance of his feelings and helps clarify the message. Another familiar and useful technique is to say what you see or what you think the patient may be feeling and let him accept or reject the explanation. You need to be ready to listen to highly charged responses if you use these approaches and to stay with the situation or see that someone else does if the patient needs to talk. Once I said to a young woman who was facing an extensive staging procedure for Hodgkin's disease, "You look sad. Do you want to tell me about it?" She did, for 45 minutes. It was a good opportunity to sort out realistic fears from unwarranted ones and to begin to order the situation in such a way that she could work with it and make decisions on a rational basis.

Patients have a right *not* to talk. We need to respect that. If we are unsure of their needs, we can ask. It is unreasonable to believe that a person will discuss personal and frightening things with a stranger, even though our professional identity gives us some credibility. It is useful to say, "Is there someone with whom you can discuss all the things that are going on?" If we are concerned that a person needs to talk, this may be pursued with him.

If his religion is important to a patient, he should have the opportunity to see his minister, priest, or rabbi as he feels this is necessary. It may also be important for family members to be involved. Spiritual counseling can be comforting, even if a person has not practiced his religion in recent years.

There are times when patients may be given too much information. The consent forms used in cancer chemotherapy protocols, as an example, spell out almost everything that could possibly happen as a result of the use of the drug. This may be an overload of information and may be upsetting, but there are positive aspects. One is that it creates an opportunity to talk about the fears the patient already experiences and to emphasize that there are benefits that should be mentioned.

It is possible to overload a person with information or to withhold needed information. To be useful in helping a patient structure his situation, facts need to be presented at a conceptual level appropriate to his understanding and to be related as much as possible to other information he has received. Family members need information if they are to join in decision making and also to help them identify the things they can do to help the patient and to reduce their own feelings of helplessness.

The last objective listed encompasses demonstrating confidence in oneself and one's ability to stay in the situation that is threatening, providing a high level of care, tolerating being with the dying patient, and doing what needs to be done. We need to clarify our objectives to stay with the person. These may include giving a specific treatment or a drug for relief of pain, helping the patient get to radiation therapy, giving intravenous fluids to relieve thirst, and listening and comforting. At the same time we may need to help the family distinguish between measures that promote comfort and those that prolong life. We may ourselves object to some of the treatment, feeling that it is unnecessary, that it is extending life when the future offers only more suffering. We need, however, to differentiate between what we feel is unnecessary treatment and treatment that seems necessary to the family so that they can say after death has occurred, "All things were done that reasonably could be done." We may confuse treatment for the sake of the family with inappropriate heroic measures, which are less often a problem as health professionals come to terms with the question of when to resuscitate and when to allow dying.

We may be with patients to give good physical care. The amount of care necessary varies with the kind of illness and the stage of illness. It is important to maintain as much mobility as possible and to keep up fluid intake even when a person has no appetite and it is not reasonable to urge him to eat. Family members may need help in deciding what interventions they can make.

I remember a petite, young half-Indian woman with whom I worked. She had advanced cervical carcinoma and had been treated with radiation therapy. She had presented at such a late stage that cure was not possible, and she had a long, uncomfortable period of dying. She was living in the home of one of her sisters and had many supportive and devoted siblings. Her husband was in jail, and she had not seen him for some time. Her three children were being taken care of by her sister. She would come to clinic and say to me, "I can't stand the way they keep looking at me; they keep fussing over me; they keep trying to make me do things." And her sister would say to me when the patient was not in the room, "I try so hard; I can't make her eat and we want her to get better. We want her to move around." It was possible to mediate and to say to the patient, "Their fussing is not picking at you. It's evidence of how much they care." It was possible to say to the family, "She's not being stubborn and rebellious. She really doesn't feel like eating, and she really has very little strength. Help her do what's possible, but if she doesn't want to eat, it is all right not to." Some of the pressure was relieved in a situation where the battling was based on love and not animosity, and she was able to be at home until two hours before she died.

A major reason for being with the patient and with the family members is to promote comfort, our own comfort as well as the comfort of the patient and family. It helps to maintain hope that is realistic. It is possible to hope that tonight will be restful, that the pain can be managed, that tomorrow can bring small things to look forward to. Patients become quite childish at times, seeking security by turning to the helping people as though they were parents. If you can help the patient structure the situation in such a way that it is manageable, he can again act as an adult.

One way to make the immediate situation more comfortable for the patient is to establish a stable environment. Keep things in the same place, do things at the same time, develop a rhythm to the day that is reassuring. Emphasize today and what is going on now and make *now* as good as possible. It supports the ego and reduces the effort needed to adapt to changes. Try to see that the people working with the dying patient are constant. By reducing the unknown and unexpected, we can reduce the feelings of helplessness. We can promote involvement in living by setting some immediate and specific goals. Such a goal may be to see the grandchildren, to go out in the yard, to have the dog in the room, to read an old favorite story, to make a quilt, or to finish a sweater. Accomplishing something helps to preserve dignity and increase self-esteem. Encouraging the patient to help with things that are appropriate to his age and position in the family may be reassuring. A woman may want most to continue her role as mother, to conceal her fears from her children because she wants to be a protector and caretaker insofar as she can. A man may be able to continue as planner in the family. He may make the major decisions. As he progresses in his adaptation and his grieving, he may be able to work with other members of the family, to pass on to them some of his duties and his knowledge. The use of reminiscence is helpful in reviewing life, in assembling the image of self that a person wishes to leave his survivors. Most people wish to leave a legacy of good memories. As you listen to a person reminiscing, you can emphasize positive things to which he refers and appreciate the good in the reconstructed life he develops.

We do much for the dying person if we help family members become involved in care to the extent that is acceptable to the patient and to them and that is consistent with the level of care needed. It also helps family to feel that they are making a contribution. We can say such things as, "It's wonderful that you can be here, and I know that it's hard for you. One of the hardest jobs we do is waiting and feeling that we're not really helping much. You are doing a great deal by being here and by being available and by listening and by caring."

The nurse is often in a position to intervene and to see that the family members who are providing for a dying patient at home have either temporary or continuing relief. The family needs to be involved in planning regularly and to know the options for care. If another level of care becomes necessary, they may need help in working out a change in such a way that they will not feel guilty. If we help with the day-to-day management of the physical and financial problems in terminal care, the patient and family may have more energy to deal with the emotional and psychological stress.

A person who is dying fears the loss of all those things that have made life worthwhile—body, family, friends, social role, self-control, identity. In addition, most people seem to fear the way of dying, possible pain, loss of control, and regression. Finally, the loneliness of death seems to be the poignant concept most difficult for all of us to face. If people close to the patient are preoccupied with their own grief and sense of outrage and loss, they may find it hard to understand the sadness and the depression of the patient. We may help them understand that anticipatory grieving can be useful to both the family and the patient as they become aware of what is going to be lost. The patient's life review will bring sadness but may also bring pleasure that can be shared with family members. At this time the family can strengthen a feeling of continuity, and the patient can get the feeling that life will continue in others, that the things he values will live on. Not everyone reaches the point where he is ready to prepare others to take over his functions or to learn his skills, but sometimes he can do some small parts of this, like acquainting a wife with the family finances or teaching a young son or daughter to manage the power mower. Relatively few people in the acute hospital setting reach the point of acceptance or resolution, unless this last admission is one of a series or the culmination of a long illness during which much of the preparatory work has been done. The people caring for a patient at home are most often involved in achieving closure.

Part of our self-acceptance involves realizing that we can rarely initiate such a process, but we need to know that wonderful changes can occur and that we help by allowing closeness and fostering communication. We are, however, more apt to be caught up in the game playing that characterizes so much of the interaction with dying people. Certainly an open awareness is the most helpful in bringing people together and allowing the real work of adaptation to begin.

A patient with whom I had been working for about eight years and with whom I had become very close died. The woman was about my age, a nurse who had breast cancer. She had had a sister who had died of breast cancer years before and believed, in spite of all the scientific information available to her, that there really was no point in any treatment. She had refused surgery when she had a small breast lump and, five years later, presented to the same physician with bilateral pleural effusions and an advanced ulcerating local breast lesion. She had had a hard time, but she had difficulty even talking about it because she felt that she had brought everything on herself and that she could not ask for any help or comfort. She told neither her husband nor her children about her problem but kept this dreadful secret to herself for five years. I asked her on her first hospitalization what she had said to her grown daughter and son, and she said, "They think I have pneumonia." After we became closer, I said to her, "I'm going to tell you something that I have never said to a patient. My mother died of breast cancer. I was with her during part of her terminal illness. I have felt badly all the years since then that we were never able to talk honestly about what was going on." She did not say anything in response to this, but when I was back two days later, her daughter was sitting on the bed. They were talking in a very intimate way that I had never seen between them before. She had dared to go through the painful process of telling her daughter what was wrong with her and what the real situation was. They cried together, and the daughter was deeply grateful that she had been treated as an adult and that they could communicate in a more honest manner. The last two years of this woman's life brought a family closeness that had never existed before.

Contrary to common fears, death is most often a peaceful event. It helps family members to stay close by if they are reassured about the nature of dying and provided with company or know that help is available. We can encourage more than one family member to share the vigil if this is possible. After death has occurred, the news should be given to a family member with others nearby to comfort and share. Each close family member should have an opportunity to see the body and say his farewell if he wishes, alone or with comforting help. If possible, the family should be given a private place to express their grief. If the physician, nurses, or other helpers have evidences of peaceful dying or messages for family members and can be available to talk about the last hours, it may help.

Another patient with inflammatory breast carcinoma died. She had lived 18 months with a difficult up-and-down course. We had been talking together during her last hospitalization when she was very cachectic and very tired. She had had soft-tissue recurrence in the abdomen and an intestinal obstruction, an emergency colostomy, and many other problems. Over the course of that year and a half she had several intensive courses of chemotherapy. We were talking about whether or not it had all been worthwhile, and she said, "Last summer was one of the greatest times in my life." She died about a day and a half after this. I had a chance to meet all four of her grown children together just after she died and to tell them about that conversation. This seemed to help in their effort to come to terms with their mother's difficult illness and vigorous treatment and their feelings that they really had not done much to help.

Even months after a death, the family members may want to talk to somebody who has known the patient and who can help them review the final illness and the things that were done. If the physician is not in a position to give the kind of review that can help in reaching a good closure, there may be other members of the health team who can.

Survivors themselves may be vulnerable. One of my graduate students was working with a young man who had acute leukemia and had been very sick, in and out of remission several times. He was the only child of elderly parents who had followed every medication and treatment during his long illness. They hoped against all odds. After he died they were distraught. I said to the student, "Make a plan so that you see the family within a week or 10 days, because they may need physical attention." She came back to me less than a week after this, rather shaken, and said, "You know, Ed's father is in the coronary care unit. He had a myocardial infarction."

Colin Parkes worked with and studied bereaved people in England and in the Boston area. He and his co-workers demonstrated that widows and widowers, within the first year after their loss, have more somatic symptoms, more need to see their physicians, and more documented illnesses than other persons of their ages do (Parkes, 1972). The loss is not just the loss of a person but the loss of a whole way of life and of most sources of satisfaction, comfort, and reassurance. The person who has lost a close family member may have a great deal of work to do to replace this member and to restructure a life that is meaningful and offers satisfaction. If grief is too prolonged, it is reasonable to suggest that the individual seek professional counseling because pathological grieving can be destructive to the individual and can immobilize him, preventing efforts to rebuild a life.

In summary, we can all play a helpful role with the dying patient and his family. We need to recognize our own limitations if we are to continue to grow in the ability to help and to risk close involvement. The nature of the physical care we offer in itself shows concern and respect. The support and openness we show families and co-workers help them contribute to a successful closure. Grief and acceptance take time, but each small success makes us better able to deal with the next dying patient and with our own losses, whenever these occur.

References

Engel, G. 1964. "Grief and Grieving." *Americal Journal of Nursing* 64:9, 93–98.

Glaser, B. G. and A. Strauss. 1965. *Awareness of Dying*. Chicago: Aldine.

Kübler-Ross, E. 1969. *On Death and Dying*. New York: Macmillan.

Lindemann, E. 1944. "Symptomatology and Management of Acute Grief." *American Journal of Psychiatry* 101:187.

Parkes, C. M. 1972. *Bereavement: Studies of Grief in Adult Life*. New York: International Universities Press.

Sudnow, D. 1967. *Passing On: The Social Organization of Dying*. Englewood Cliffs, N.J.: Prentice-Hall.

❧❧❧ 5

The Nurse and Home Care of the Terminally Ill

Virginia G. Wessells

The topic at hand is a broad one. I intend to convey concern with the physio-psychosocial states of the terminal patient, his family, and the environment for his care. I must also make some statement about what nursing is and about what the nurse has to do with care of the terminally ill cancer patient at home.

My philosophy of client care is holistic. Mankind's various states cannot be separated into physiological, psychological, or social, although the immediate problem may fall into one of those areas. A broken toe is primarily a physical ailment, but the pain, disability, and loss of independence suffered as a result have important psychological, social and perhaps economic consequences. The patient's and family's ability to cope, support, and use existing resources or discover new resources may be crucial to obtaining or maintaining healthy states for one and all. Putting a cast on the foot may be essential, but it can also be attending to the "least" of this patient's ailments. It may be compared to suturing and applying a bandage to the slashed wrists of a suicidal patient and assuming that "everything will be all right" because the patient has been treated for his most pressing and visible problem. The same parallel can be drawn when we assume that the dying person will be just fine if appropriate physical care, equipment, and a beautiful environment are provided but we ignore the patient's and family's need to share and cope with their grief and grieving reactions. No one will deny that casts and bandages have their place as long as we give equal weight to and concern for the psychosocial needs of the patient. Can we legitimately say that we are providing "health care" unless we do this? I think not, and I hope my practice reflects this belief.

I believe that nursing is a public service that provides health care to individuals in a holistic frame of reference (client-centered care). Nurses today are educated to be generalists so that, at graduation from a baccalaureate program, they have learned the basic information needed to assist the client(s) to maintain health, prevent illness and adverse happenings, and restore health as well. We all grant that the new graduate needs additional practice and learning to be adept and skillful in both general and specialty areas of practice. Fortunately, programs of various kinds are being tried out to enable her to do this. These efforts should continue, for in my opinion the greatest value the nurse has today in our complex health care system is her ability to function both as a skillful generalist and specialist and to be involved in the physical, psychological, and social areas of care. Recent studies in use of the nurse in expanded roles have shown that, with little additional knowledge, she can undertake a much higher level of independent practice in all areas of care than anyone previously believed. If only to reduce fragmentation of care, one of her most important services to clients and families at this time may be her knowledge and skill in "keeping the parts glued together" and in helping clients to preserve their rights within the health care system. I believe that nursing cuts across the functions of many other disciplines at this time and that this condition will probably continue far into the future. The accuracy of this view has not been tested by research, but I hope it will be. For the present then, nursing should continue to prepare nurses as generalists, enlarging their knowledge appropriately in both physical and psychosocial areas, and encouraging the development of specialization through additional education and clinical practice.

Table 5.1. Three Frames of Reference for Nurse Function in Care of the Terminally Ill at Home

Maintenance	Prevention	Restoration
Assisting the client to obtain or maintain those requirements basic to health	Input, direction, and management of client care so that unnecessary, unsafe, painful, or dangerous events, situations, or circumstances are avoided or amended	Assistance with modification of the client/family condition or situation to restore the highest level of independent function possible

Food   Elimination
Drink   Cleanliness
Sleep   Warmth
         Oxygen
Sexual fulfillment
Safety
Comfort
Exercise and weight bearing
Meaningful activity
Diversion
Social interaction
Love
Self-acceptance
Self-esteem
Body image
Status
Recognition
Self-actualization
Knowledge about:
  self
    Present health status
    Future possibilities
  Environment
    Helping persons
    Other resources
	Nutritional deficit
	Contamination of food and drink
	Dehydration
	Electrolyte imbalance
	Sustained loss of sleep
	Inadequate, difficult, or painful
	  elimination
	Excesses of heat and cold
	Infections and irritations
	Pathological states
	Bone fracture
	Bone demineralization
	Muscle atrophy, loss of strength
	Joint contractures
	Sensory loss
	Sensory deprivation
	Loss of self-esteem
	Reduction of independence and
	  self-care ability
	Emotional depression—confusion
	Ignorance of health state and
	  individual rights
	Excessive stress
	Unsafe equipment, environment,
	  or activity
		Physiological imbalance
		  or altered function
		Heal wounds or fractures
		  and irritations
		Increase muscle strength
		Improve range of joint
		  motion
		Increase ambulation and
		  activity level
		Improve independence in
		  activities of daily living

Table 5.1 defines the three major areas of nursing function in client care and illustrates their scope for nursing practice in the home care of terminally ill adults. I acknowledge that my beliefs have been particularly influenced by Henderson (1966, p. 15), who believes that "The unique function of the nurse is to assist the individual, sick or well, in the performance of those activities contributing to health, or its recovery (or to a peaceful death) that he would perform unaided if he had the necessary strength, will or knowledge." The conceptual model of Abdellah et al. (1960; 1965) and the works of other nurse

scholars have also made impact on the selected frames of reference used in the table. Credit is also due Maslow (1954), who was the first to identify a hierarchy of human needs. The adaptation shown is my invention and was influenced by many other authors who have made additions to and adaptations of Maslow's model.

The following examples illustrate how nurse function may differ in the three categories. If we say that a basic need of all persons is for food, then the nurse has maintenance functions to perform. She could carry out functions (depending on the particular patient's problems) such as:

1. assisting the client to get food stamps for purchase of food by informing him of places to go,
2. feeding the patient who cannot feed himself,
3. cutting up food, opening cartons, and arranging food in the tray for a patient with disabling rheumatoid arthritis who feeds himself but cannot carry out the identified activities.

In a preventive frame of reference, to prevent nutritional deficit she could:

1. identify nutritional deficit through analysis of patient's food intake with intent to act for correction,
2. contact the social worker to obtain money for supplementary liquid feedings to improve the nutritional status of the terminal patient with cancer of the esophagus,
3. administer the feeding to a patient who is too weak to do an adequate job of feeding himself.

In a restorative frame of reference, she could restore physiological imbalance by:

1. administering intravenous fluids with insulin (through doctor's order) to correct for hyperglycemia in the client with ketoacidosis,
2. assist the patient to plan for changes in diet to correct the hyperglycemia of diabetes mellitus,
3. plan and assist with the execution of a bowel training regimen for an incontinent patient.

I contend that the nurse's role largely consists of maintenance and prevention if executed at an acceptable professional level. Woe to the nurse who works in settings where restorative or administrative requirements usurp all of her time and effort. In such circumstances patients become dehydrated and constipated; develop bedsores, inappropriate behavior patterns, and loss of self-esteem; learn little about their conditions and the treatments they are being given; and accrue many other unnecessary adverse effects for lack of maintenance and prevention.

The patient with cancer is likely to encounter the nurse and receive services from her along the entire continuum of care as he experiences diagnostic and restorative services and a therapeutic regimen. As the most numerous of the health care personnel, the nurse is present in almost every phase of health care, including that in the physician's office, ambulatory care settings, hospitals, nursing homes, diagnostic and treatment centers, and home care. The description that follows is based on the hospital as the first point of contact—a parallel to the situation in which our rehabilitation project personnel function.

Phase 1. In the hospital care of the patient with cancer the nurse finds that her role is dependent and complementary to that of the physician, as well as to numerous other health disciplines. She plans and gives direct nursing care, directs others in giving care, and implements medical regimens. She plays an important teaching role, varying from orientating the patient to the unit, preoperative and postoperative teaching, interpreting testing, administering health care regimens, giving medications, and making resources available. She does much coordinating of care with other disciplines both in and out of the hospital and promotes referrals to appropriate individuals and agencies.

Phase 2. The patient is discharged home with a referral to the public health nurse (if needed). Acting on orders from the physician who signed the referral, the home care nurse takes over. She assesses the patient and his environment and identifies the prevailing problems (some of which have been missed on the referral) and makes independent decisions about the client's care based on mutual agreements with the client or family or both. She does health counseling, teaches, and assists patient and family to find and mobilize resources.

She acts as liaison with other disciplines and agencies by various means—through direct contact, as well as written and verbal communications. She implements the physician's orders and gives direct care as well.

Phase 3. The patient returns to the clinic or doctor's office to get medical checkup or therapy or both. The clinic nurse participates in assessment of the patient's family's overall needs, teaches, counsels, may administer therapy (chemotherapy and other), refers, helps obtain resources, and maintains close liaison with the physician and other available disciplines to plan and execute effective care and solve ongoing problems. She may communicate new orders and other changes in the health care regimen to the home care nurse.

Phase 4. Treatment continues over an undetermined period with successful or unsuccessful outcomes. During this period both home care nurse and clinic nurse have an important role to play in establishing a relationship with the patient and the family so that progress may be made in meeting the patient's and family's needs for acceptance of the disease and its implications for the future and in assisting them to deal with the grief stages if the disease is uncontrolled or has disfiguring effects. During this period all the health care professionals and their assistants should be helping to assist the client to achieve the highest level of return of normal function and activity level as is possible within the limits of the disabling effects of the disease and therapy.

Phase 5. The uncontrolled-disease group begin to decline into the terminal phase of the disease. In this phase, maintenance and preventive regimens move to the forefront once more. The nurse teaches family and patient ways to handle declining physical abilities and to maintain the highest level of the activities of daily living (ADL) as is possible (or she may give support to physical therapy, occupational therapy, and recreation therapy programs designed for the patient). She provides counseling in physiological maintenance regimens with appropriate input from the physician. Beneficial psychosocial consequences result in parallel with the emotional support she provides by:

Psychosocial consequence

Meeting physiological needs and preventing adverse happenings.	Reduces stress, promotes comfort and safety.
Paying attention to patient and family, by meeting physiological needs, by listening, reflecting, discussing, counseling, referring to appropriate persons to meet psychosocial needs, as well as other needs.	Establishes trust relationship, promotes positive mental health, meets patient/family needs for status and recognition.
Being consistent, truthful, and helpful.	Promotes trust relationship and positive mental health.
Promoting and supporting highest level of independent function possible within patient's physio-psychosocial limitations.	Promotes self-acceptance and self-esteem, maintains body image and adaptive process.
Assessing the patient's level of acceptance of this disease and readiness to move to another stage. Intervenes or assists by planning intervention with others.	Meets learning needs. Modifies behavior for positive acceptance of self and acceptability to others.
Giving appropriate feedback to patient about his performance, encouraging a positive outlook.	Promotes belief in self and increases confidence in self's potential to do whatever needs to be done in coping with the demands or stress.

This list is not intended to be exhaustive, but it illustrates some of the very important actions that nurses (as well as other health care providers) engage in that may assist the patient and family throughout the period of care. As the patient approaches death, one would hope that he has adjusted to his impending death and made appropriate plans that the family can accept. Ideally the grieving process is well on the way and emotional control prevails so that appropriate effort and support can be invested in the patient's physical care, comfort, and safety needs. If this is not so, the nurse or others may be instrumental in obtaining the necessary counseling or, in some instances, act as counselor.

The teaching role of the nurse increases where the patient or family have had little experience with the care of bedridden or helpless persons. Food, drink, elimination, personal hygiene, mouth care, comfort measures, use of equipment and devices for comfort and preventive care, and control of pain often become paramount issues as the patient becomes less and less competent in self-care. The prevention of skin breakdown, infection, constipation, bone demineralization, malnutrition and dehydration are crucial for comfort and appropriate maintenance care. The nurse monitors medications and the patient's responses to them and acts as liaison with the physician and pharmacist. The nurse gives direct care along with family or other caregivers.

The following case example illustrates the care of a terminal cancer patient.

Mrs. M. was first encountered during her hospitalization for diagnostic workup of severe weakness of her lower extremities and pain on ambulation. The patient had been treated for several years by a local physician for cancer of the thyroid. He referred her to a medical oncologist on the staff of our institution when she exhibited the symptoms of paraparesis. She was found to have metastasis to the T-11 and T-12 vertebrae with collapse and spinal cord compression. She was treated by a decompression laminectomy and fitted with a Jewett brace and later transferred to the department of physical medicine and rehabilitation, where she received extended treatment to restore her to maximum functional level. She was discharged home able to do self-care at the wheelchair level.

The Cancer Rehabilitation Project accepted home care referral on Mrs. M. with aims to:

1. evaluate her environment and assist her in making adjustment and adapting ADL at the wheelchair level,
2. promote exercise programs designed to strengthen the upper extremities and to improve transfer ability from bed to wheelchair and commode,
3. promote independence in ambulation if feasible,
4. provide emotional support and assistance in the grief process to patient and family as the need becomes apparent.

Initial assessment by the team members at home included evaluation of the physical strength and activity level by physical and occupational therapists, evaluation for maintenance and preventive nursing care needs by the nursing coordinator, exploration of financial resources and need for help in locating a sitter to assist with patient's maintenance care by the social worker, and assessment by all the team members (during contact) of the patient's and family's present emotional state and need for counseling assistance.

The plan for care that evolved used primarily the physical therapist, occupational therapist, and the rehabilitation aide assigned to the continuing care team. The exercise and training programs and monitoring of patient's maintenance care were implemented over a period of several months. After an initial home care visit the nurse coordinator saw Mrs. M. in our tumor clinic when she came for evaluation and chemotherapy. The nursing coordinator gave direction to the aide in nursing matters—otherwise, the aide was directed and supervised by the physical therapist and the occupational therapist.

During the next three months the patient achieved independence in transfer from bed to wheelchair and engaged in some cooking and light housekeeping tasks. She did not achieve ambulation but worked diligently toward this end.

Disaster struck midway in her fourth month of home care when she suddenly regressed and became unable to stand independently and transfer. A subsequent neurological examination revealed that the metastasis of the disease in her spine had attacked the vertebrae above the T-10 level, and she now also had lesions in the ribs, sacrum, and lungs.

The patient was told about the new discoveries. She at first denied the information and moved through several very trying behavioral processes in the fifth and sixth months of home care.

Her physical condition deteriorated to complete paraplegia and sensory loss below the T-10 level. She developed tachycardia and moderately severe edema of her body below the T-10 level and especially in her lower extremities. She became incontinent of bladder and bowel and had bladder spasms. She was physically unable to participate in physical or occupational therapy programs, and these therapists came to act only as consultants to the nurse in her care.

Mrs. M.'s family members struggled to make some difficult decisions about who should give her care and whether or not she could continue chemotherapy. The nurse acted as direct caregiver, taught family and sitter to give care, planned maintenance programs, and counseled the family about when to seek medical care for the patient. She assisted the family in obtaining the information needed to decide about continuance of the chemotherapy and further treatment. At present the nurse is managing the patient's care by liaison with the clinic physician in harmony with the patient/family decision to stop therapy and do all care for the patient at home until her death. The rehabilitation aide continues to visit and assists the nurse with supervision and direction of Mrs. M.'s care.

The emotional struggle of the patient to accept death and the dying process has involved the nurse, more so because the family have been unable to talk with the patient about her feelings. In the early stages the nurse and sitter were the only ones who would listen to Mrs. M's expressions of fear and allow her to explore her feelings. Intervention at a crucial point by the patient counselor on our rehabilitation team has been invaluable. He has counseled husband and patient and is now involved with other family members as well. He has, moreover, assisted the nurse as she felt the need to explore her own decisions and interactions with the patient.

Mrs. M. appears to have made much progress toward acceptance of her imminent death, but help is still needed. The family cannot yet talk with her about death and will continue to receive counseling.

In summary I believe that the nurse presently plays a major role in management and execution of care of the terminally ill at home and has potential for increasing her usefulness through expansion of role by additional education and experience. Initially nurses must seek to document their current practice in home care of the terminally ill and then promulgate means to expand their role as it is appropriate for effectiveness, efficiency, and increased satisfaction of patients and their families.

References

Abdellah, F. G. et al. 1960. *Patient Centered Approaches to Nursing*. New York: Macmillan.

Abdellah, F. G. and E. Levine. 1965. *Better Patient Care Through Nursing Research*. New York: Macmillan.

Henderson, V. 1966. *The Nature of Nursing*. New York: Macmillan.

Maslow, A. 1954. *Motivation and Personality*. New York: Harper.

ꙮꙮꙮ 6

Home Care of the Cancer Patient

Isadore Rossman

M any stock phrases, however banal, that describe the home must mirror important feelings. "There is no place like home," and "Home Sweet Home" are judgmental declarations pointing to a meaningful superiority of the home. Although, when vertical mobility changes an individual's values and life-style, the place of the home is altered, generally speaking a whole constellation of positive values and feelings remains attached to the home. In the symbols of psychoanalysis, home is equated with the mother figure. "All the comforts of home" is an advertising phrase designed to seduce us to an unknown spot. "Home is where the bread is blessed," and "Home cooking" delineate aspects of orality and ingestion. Profound attachment to the home extends from one end of the lifespan to the other. The young child races home after school as to a haven for respite. Old people cling to their homes and resist transfer to other environments with a fierceness and tenacity that sometimes seem irrational. But validation for all this stubbornness is clear when confusion and intellectual decompensation occur after the transfer. As for those in neither extreme, however much we may enjoy a succession of new experiences and sights, as in travel, sooner or later we weary of them and gladly return to home base. As one considers the pro-

60

found values of the home in normal development, it becomes pertinent to inquire into their weight and applicability to the individual stricken with cancer.

Over the past quarter century on our home care program we have had more than 800 patients with cancer. This has given us opportunity to observe the patient both in hospital and home environments and thus compare the impact of these two settings. Admittedly one variable over this time are changes that have occurred in attitudes toward cancer. Twenty-five years ago the diagnosis was seldom discussed with the patient, and conspiracies of silence were often maintained by both family and doctor. Families frequently told us that, for one or another valid reason, as, for example, a "long illness" in another member of the family, knowledge of the diagnosis should be withheld. This point of view often coincided with that held by the patient. The patient generally knew, or suspected, the existence of cancer and, by what has been termed the schizoid maneuver, pushed it out of consciousness. Improvements in treatment and a new willingness to recognize and discuss the disease are modifying previous points of view considerably, though some of the reasons for concealment still exist. Inoperable cancer, for which irradiation or chemotherapy is not indicated, still presents a singularly grave emotional challenge to the patient, the caring relatives, and the doctor. The challenge is even greater in the home setting than in the hospital. The patient in the hospital is generally in for some positive maneuver, whereas this is seldom the case at home. Home care thus resolves itself into a major challenge in the care and maintenance of an obviously dying cancer patient. Not all patients and all families are equal to this. Hence, experience has dictated the need for admissions criteria into such a home care program.

Traditionally on our program a two-phase evaluation is performed (Cherkasky, Rossman, and Rogatz, 1961). The first, done by the physician, identifies whether the patient is medically suitable for home care. When close medical monitoring, intravenous therapy, or major round-the-clock needs exist, the patient is not suitable. We have, however, had many patients who have had blood transfusions at home, who have had thoracenteses and paracenteses, and for whom courses of chemotherapy with dosages monitored by blood counts have been successfully managed in the home setting. We have taught family members to give injections of narcotics and perform various skilled nursing procedures at home. It is clear from our experience that complex programs of care can be transferred into the home setting with treatment regimens maintained at a high level by doctor, nurse, and family jointly (Rossman, 1954). A certain kind of experience is necessary to make correct medical judgments about which cancer patient can go home. It is unfortunate and sometimes traumatic to accept a patient on home care inexpertly, only to have him sent back to the hospital within a short time.

But even more important than the medical judgment is the social judgment, which calls for empathy and perceptiveness on the part of the social worker (Rossman and Kissick, 1961). After the patient has been judged medically acceptable, the social worker has next to determine whether the patient and family can make a go of it at home. There are more rejections for social than for medical reasons on our program. Because of the trying nature of the care of some terminal cancer patients, the family members involved must have interpersonal resources, endurance, and strengths. Again, it is unnecessarily traumatic and even a major blunder to misjudge this and have the patient sent home only to return bewildered and depressed to the hospital. A solid, well-grounded relationship between the patient and other members of the family is a necessary base for home care. When family relationships are hostile or shallow, the demands of home care may be shattering.

It is an old truism on our program that the test of a good marriage is adverse circumstances rather than normal ones. Complex situations may exist in reality. Thus, one may ponder numerous intrafamiliar factors and weigh many pros against many cons. A daughter may be willing to care for a mother who is sick, disoriented, and incontinent, but this may be at some cost to her own children. Family members sometimes go on and on in a deteriorating situation, expending all their strengths in an exhausting day and night "on call" program. It may be wise in such circumstances for the doctor or social worker to stress the validity of alternatives. When, however, selection criteria are favorable, home care of the cancer patient has uniquely positive values for both patient and family of an order not apparent to those who deal only with hospital care.

Home care is a good deal more economical than hospital care, and documentation exists that home care programs save needed hospital beds or cut down on the duration of hospitalization (Cherkasky, Rossman, and Rogatz, 1961). Recent formidable rises in the cost of a hospital day have emphasized anew the cost-effectiveness of alternatives. But financial considerations are not the dominant ones for contemplating extension of organized home care to cancer patients. In a completely affluent society with all cost considerations relegated to limbo, medical care in the home setting would not go by the board. Especially for the cancer patient, there are many persuasive reasons for emphasizing home rather than institutional care. Cancer encompasses a number of disease entities and a wide spectrum of disability. Some of them inevitably lead to a homebound status. Because of variability in the way in which the sequence evolves, little change may occur over considerable periods of time. This has been illustrated repeatedly in some of our patients who were homebound for years. Sometimes one can plot a course marked by a burst of therapeutic activity, such as irradiation, chemotherapy, or hormonal therapy, followed by protracted periods of partial improvement or illness plateaus. If palliative measures continue to improve and multiply, while the "cure" escapes us, that segment of the illness for which home care is applicable will in fact continue to grow. This would lead to enlarged and continued demands for medical and nursing care, for more planning and counseling from social workers, and for more in the way of recreational and diversional measures. With such developments the number of needed institutional beds, if that were to be the answer, would be huge, but as the experience of home care programs indicates, prolonged institutional care would be, for many reasons, an inferior alternative to home care. Cancer makes many of its victims ill, helpless, or dependent for long periods of time, and planning must address itself to this phase of the disease, not to the active therapeutic bursts alone.

Many observations comparing the impact of the hospital as against the home indicate the many positive functions of the home setting. The weight of home factors is often unsuspected by hospital personnel, who observe a rate of decline and project it into a prognosis. It then comes as a considerable surprise to find that the rate of decline can be modified and that a favorable alteration can be of impressive magnitude. Patients who have been losing weight and strength and whose capacities have declined reverse all these when transferred into the home setting. Some of the factors responsible for such improvement are apparent to the home observer. Improvement in weight and strength occurs, not only because radiation and other noxious therapies cease, but also because the home supplies a catering diet attuned to the patient's wants, in a manner that no hospital kitchen can match. Stimuli toward mobility become more apparent in the home setting. Thus, the cancer patient may elect to eat at the family table rather than at a bedside tray or choose to walk to the bathroom rather than be washed in bed. Numerous similar contrasts occur throughout the day.

It is simply a fact that the modern hospital cannot mobilize emotional supportive resources for the cancer patient, and, almost inevitably, it continues to be a threatening or unpleasant setting (Rossman, Clarke, and Rudnick, 1962). The cancer patient may be subjected to painful or nauseating treatments, may be incised and mutilated. He is exposed to the ministrations of strangers, many preoccupied or abstracted, who are shifted at eight-hour intervals. Hospital routines and regimens are utterly beyond the patient's control or veto; hence, the sense of powerlessness is increased. There are noises, mostly unpleasant, and the alarums and excursions of such events as cardiac arrests. Such frequent and repeated procedures as drawing blood are perceived by many a patient as a withdrawal of his strength or a diminution of his reserves. After many days or weeks of this, it is easy to see why the cancer patient may see his transfer home as the lifting of a threat and a deliverance. The contrasts in the home are obvious. The noises, threats, and attacks of the hospital environment and its undefined periphery where the operating rooms and cobalt machines lurk are replaced by an environment that is encapsulated, and familiar and, indeed, one in which the patient may assume control and in which family members become reliable aides. Not to be neglected in the comparisons is that the cancer patient returned to home may well be able to assume old role relationships. Even if bedridden, a mother may still enact maternal roles—an important change over the loss of role and functions imposed by the hospital bed.

It is unfortunate that in the United States most cancer patients who are ill at home do not get comprehensive care. Indeed, most medical practitioners tend to make the care delivered in this setting somewhat skimpy. Some practitioners perceive the terminal cancer patient at home as having largely passed beyond their province and conclude that calls on such a patient are unnecessary. A contrasting view, as exemplified by our program, emphasizes the many reasons why it is just these circumstances that call for visiting. The advantages of the home as a therapeutic environment can become manifest only when a reasonable number of resources are marshaled into the home environment. What the optimum number of such home-delivered services would be has never been fully explored, since home care programs labor generally under a burden of inadequate financing and resources. At one time on our program when personnel were more readily available, there were, in addition to the basic team of doctor, nurse, and social worker, recreational and work therapists; and when nursing needs progressed, student nurses were supplied as often as every day. Heavy nursing burdens are now being met through such community agencies as the New York City Division of the American Cancer Society and Cancer Care. But the keystone in the arch is an indoctrinated caring relative whose qualitative and quantitative contributions can be quite astonishing.

Perhaps the most noteworthy change produced by home care is the message transmitted by this mobilization of resources. It states that the dying cancer patient is worthy of effort, time, and coordinated energies and thus negates any previous formulation that the patient has passed beyond the point where such effort is indicated. The impact on the family is equally great. One of the doleful moods frequently seen in such homes derives from the feeling that the family has been abandoned by the community to carry an increasingly heavy burden alone. In addition, there are myriad practical difficulties. How can one get a doctor to make a house call? How can one get a more comfortable bed? How can one have nursing services daily? Can homemaking needs be supplied? Is there any help when financial resources are pinched? All of the oppressive implications of these queries are resolved by our professionals. The immediate effect of coming onto home care is thus to relieve the family of these unnecessary burdens and free them to give more to the cancer patient. It is apparent that the transformation of the home environment described here is of a different order of magnitude from what exists when only a doctor, however devoted, makes home calls. As an example, for years, visitors to our program were astonished to have an advanced cancer patient described in clinical detail and then walk into the home and see a cheerful patient painting or even doing light work for pay. Those who consider the tragedies of human existence noteworthy, may consider the implications of a cancer patient's finding that he has artistic talent only after coming onto a home care program.

As an example of the transformation of the home, the following case history of one of our earlier myeloma patients is illustrative (Rossman, 1956). In addition to detailing an eight-year course on our program, it points up the folly of prognostication with cancer patients, for this patient was thought to be moribund at the time of referral:

I.J., 53 years old, was on our program for eight years, had multiple myeloma, and was referred to us after a laminectomy occasioned by collapse of several thoracic vertebrae and cord compression. He was placed in a body cast and discharged to the home care program completely bedridden. He was seriously ill with widespread osteolytic lesions, severe anemia, radiculitis, and recurrent pneumonitis.

Medical. During his first year on the program, 102 visits were made by physicians and medical consultants. He received numerous transfusions, required large doses of narcotics, and the prognosis was poor. After a year of intensive treatment, his hemoglobin dropped below 6 grams, and increasing hyperglobulinemia was noted. During a considerable part of that year, the patient had recurrent carbuncles and furuncles treated at home with antibiotics and incision and drainage. After three years on home care, spontaneous improvement occurred. The anemia disappeared, and there was no further progression of myelomatous lesions. The femoral lesions were so extensive as to prohibit ambulation. During the eight years he was on home care, the patient had eight readmissions to the hospital; several of the early ones were for radiotherapy for relief of pain, one was for breaking of morphine addiction, and another for extraction of remaining teeth and making of dentures. He died in hospital after a prolonged downhill course.

Social. Throughout this period, the patient's care had come largely from a devoted wife. After instruction by the visiting nurse service, she assumed a large part of the nursing burden for this bedridden patient. During the first two years, when the patient was visibly failing, she was frequently depressed. She was given psychologic aid by a case worker with whom a warm friendship developed. The relationship was extremely supportive during periods of grief and despair. The many problems involved in the husband's illness, including changes in his medical status, were frequently discussed. Financial problems were particularly troublesome, since only marginal support came from two married daughters.

At the suggestion of the social worker, one room was rented out; the income from this was helpful. After several years, arrangements were made for the family to receive financial assistance from the Department of Welfare. Turning to the welfare agency represented a crisis to both wife and daughters, all of whom initially rejected the plan with strong feelings of shame at "accepting charity." The plan was finally worked out with them in a persuasive and supportive manner. This relieved the wife of one of her major burdens.

Nursing. For the first three years on the program, three visits, averaging about one hour, were made each week. General nursing care, including enemas, changes of dressings, and parenteral administration of drugs, was given. A nurse assisted at transfusions and various minor surgical procedures. The wife was instructed in bedside nursing care, the giving of hypodermics, and the like; under supervision she became quite expert.

Physiotherapy. The patient received physiotherapy for a nine-month period. This was directed toward getting the patient, who had been bedridden for more than four years, into better physical condition. Active and passive exercise was employed, plus heat treatment and massage. A spinal brace was constructed, and the patient was finally able to get out of bed and into a wheelchair by himself. This was a great advance, since, for the first time in five years, he could be taken out of doors.

Occupational therapy was modified at various times by the vicissitudes of his illness and by his changing interests and disinterests. It was largely recreational. Initially it was adapted to a weak, bedridden patient whose physical capacity was quickly exhausted. Later, as he was out of bed, more elaborate procedures were added, such as weaving. The patient was visited at intervals of approximately three weeks.

As the disease progresses, the needs increase, and the physical and psychological demands may become heavier. Our policy is to increase our support in parallel fashion by supplying more help, visits, nursing, or housekeeping aid. This diminishes the patient's feeling that he is becoming too much of a burden or wearing the family down. The family that wants to care for a sick member at home should not be physically exhausted as a result of that decision. In a few instances we have had a home declared to be a foster home and thereby enabled the Bureau of Social Services of this city to pay a monthly stipend to the caring relatives. Though many families are not poor enough to qualify for this, or if poor enough, too proud to do so, a routine subsidy would represent an interesting new approach. We could state to the family that the magnitude of their day-and-night help merits recognition from the disbursing authorities who would otherwise pay out much larger sums for hospital and nursing home care.

Should dying occur in the home? Since our home care program has always had an unassailable right to readmit to the hospital, alternatives are always open to the physician in attendance. The answer has to be individualized in terms of the physician's judgment and knowledge of patient and family. Some families have incorporated the facts into their thinking, have made their peace with the inevitable, and accept a terminal situation that includes dehydration and perhaps a slowly progressive coma. Other families, who have never been willing to accept the disheartening facts, fight strenuously for every day of life. With them, returning the patient to the hospital may be a desired solution. The patient's point of view is by no means to be disregarded. He may assent or dissent. Very often, the patient has become quite passive, and the decisions are made by family and physician. Social and cultural factors play a role so that generalizations do not apply. Obviously in a family grouping in which death at home has been culturally acceptable, as among the Irish with their traditional wake, such a background may play an important role in decision making. Religion may also be decisive. The Catholic patient may be willing to receive the last rites at home and die there. In a discussion regarding this with one Catholic nurse I was told, "We regard death as a pause, not as the end. Death is more like a comma in the middle of a sentence than a period at the end.''

Some families, however, stand in terror of death or believe, albeit irrationally, that the hospital may deal with it better or somehow prolong life. In such circumstances the moribund cancer patient is transferred out of his home. Both in relation to this final phase and to all that precedes it, it is clear that the role of the physician is to weigh multiple factors in a broadly humanitarian framework.

References

Cherkasky, M., I. Rossman, and P. Rogatz. 1961. *Guide to Organized Home Care*, p. 34. Chicago: Hospital Research and Educational Trust.

Rossman, I. 1954. "Treatment of Cancer on a Home Care Program." *Journal of the American Medical Association* 156:827–30.

Rossman, I. 1956. "Suitability of Home Care for the Cancer Patient." *Geriatrics* 11:407–12.

Rossman, I., M. Clarke, and B. Rudnick. 1962. "Total Rehabilitation in a Home Care Setting." *New York State Journal of Medicine* 62:1215–19.

Rossman, I. and W. L. Kissick. 1961. "Home Care and the Cancer Patient." American Cancer Society Symposium, "Total Care of the Cancer Patient," pp. 161–69.

How Group Meetings Ease
the Stress of Cancer on Patients
and Their Families

M. L. S. Vachon, W. A. L. Lyall, and H. Pollack

Many of the problems experienced by patients and families involved with life-threatening illness develop early in the course of the
disease (Vachon, 1972; Lyall et al., 1973; Vachon and Lyall, 1976;
Vachon et al., 1976; Rogers and Vachon, 1975). In our present zeal
to improve the care of the terminally ill, we often work against insurmountable odds because we are intervening too late. Frequently, by
the time a patient is diagnosed as being terminal, his relationships
with family, friends, and physician have deteriorated considerably,
he is stripped of his sense of control over his own destiny, and he
responds with tremendous depression, fear, and anger.

His response is certainly understandable, and yet, if someone
had intervened earlier, perhaps some of his difficulties could have
been alleviated, if not eliminated. For example, a young man was admitted to hospital for what he expected was minor surgery. When he
awoke, the surgeon said "I had to do a lot more than I expected, but
it would be worse if you were a woman." His wife was told over the

phone, "You'll have to come and see what your husband looks like now that he has had surgery." No one spoke to this couple about the reason for surgery, the diagnosis and its implications, or the effect it might have on their marriage.

Gradually the relationship began to deteriorate. The couple was eventually told the husband had cancer and was in the terminal phase of his disease. They were referred for counseling, for they were considering separation.

Frequent exposure to such situations caused one of us (M. V.) to wonder what could be done to intervene more effectively with patients and families in the early stages of their illness to alleviate some of the later problems. As an outgrowth of this concern, weekly group meetings were begun at the Princess Margaret Hospital Lodge, which is a 57-bed unit for outpatients from outside Toronto who are receiving radiotherapy treatment at Princess Margaret Hospital. Groups were co-led by the head nurse at the lodge (Mrs. Patricia Walker) and one of the authors (M. V.) The groups were attended by patients who were newly diagnosed and by those receiving active treatment for recurrence of their disease. Whenever possible, family members were encouraged to attend.

The groups provided patients in the initial phase of their illness with an opportunity to share their fears, clarify their misconceptions, and improve their coping skills. Here they were encouraged to express their feelings of fear, isolation, depression, and anger. They gained understanding, acceptance, and support for these feelings from other group members. In addition, the "more experienced" cancer patients were able to offer suggestions for living with the stigma of cancer, overcoming the fear of family and friends, and coping with the panic so often associated with their new diagnosis. Patients were helped to verbalize their questions, such as, "Why did this happen to me?" "Will my children catch or inherit my cancer?" "What will happen to me now that I have this terrible disease?" and "Is there anything I can do to save myself?"

Frequently, newly diagnosed patients are angry at their primary physician. He may be accused of misinterpreting presenting symptoms, delaying the diagnosis, or even causing the cancer. Whereas much of this anger may be projection, the patient must nonetheless work through the anger, for he will be returning to the physician for followup care. In addition, the patient is helped to improve communication with the oncologist by letting the doctor know how much information he, the patient, wants about his disease. Patients share their differences openly in this area; some want to know nothing more than when to come for their next treatment, while others want to know detailed information regarding their disease and its treatment. We cannot presume to decide for patients what they should know; we help them make their own decisions in this matter with much group support.

Throughout the group meetings and in the supportive milieu of the lodge, patients are encouraged to assume independence, take responsibility for dealing with their disease and its treatment, improve their coping skills, and try to understand that their attitude can affect the outcome of their illness, at least to some degree. In this way it is hoped that patients will not assume the passive, helpless attitude that may lead to interference with treatment and/or premature death from cancer.

As an outgrowth of the lodge groups, a similar program was initiated on two inpatient units, as well as for parents of children with cancer. To date, more than 2,000 patients and family members have attended these meetings. They claim that the sessions have answered their questions, decreased their anxiety, provided them with alternative coping skills, and enabled them to gain hope from meeting other cancer patients. Some have gone on to develop similar programs in the home communities. These groups approach newly diagnosed patients who are coming to Princess Margaret Hospital and help to allay their anxiety. As a result we now see significantly less fear in the out-of-town patients being admitted to the lodge and the hospital.

Aware of the success of the program and concerned that more of its benefits were not available to Toronto residents, the Toronto unit of the Canadian Cancer Society approached the authors to develop a pilot project and start such programs for local residents.

After much thought it was decided that for maximum benefit we would begin a training program for professionals already involved with cancer patients in local hospitals and the community. It was hoped that in this way the agencies would commit themselves to improving care for cancer patients and their families through the use of such unstructured group meetings. Most of the 18 enrolled in the course to become group leaders are nurses, although we also have one social worker and one radiotherapy technologist. The initial part of the course ran for two hours weekly for ten weeks. This was followed by individual supervision in group experiences, and then the group reassembled for continuing group supervision.

The model we are using attempts to give people a chance to attend these groups at many different points in the illness. Groups in some of the hospitals are primarily for newly diagnosed patients and families. Other groups focus on those receiving chemotherapy for recurrent disease, and two others serve patients receiving palliative treatment. With this model people get their immediate questions answered by the staff responsible for their care and share their concerns with others going through the same experience.

At one such meeting ten women receiving chemotherapy for recurrent breast disease shared their feelings about their initial diagnosis. Many had entered surgery with reassurance that their lump was benign. They talked of looking at the clock while receiving anesthesia thinking that they would be able to tell by the time they woke up whether or not they had cancer. None were helped when they awoke hours later to deal with their initial shock. Most felt they adjusted well, however, having been reassured that their cancer had been removed and all would be well. When many developed bone pain several months later, they ignored it or treated it as arthritis—seeing no connection between that and their mastectomy. When they eventually sought medical treatment, they were shocked to realize this was bony metastases. Recurrence was a major problem for most of them and a far greater shock than their initial diagnosis.

Comparing symptoms, they could see that some in the group had really profited from chemotherapy. One woman said she had been paralyzed and told she had only six months to live. When her doctor was on holidays, she was in great pain, and so a friend called another physician, who started her on chemotherapy. One and one-half years later she appeared to be well on maintenance chemotherapy.

Many spoke of living for today and enjoying as much as possible. They shared ideas about setting priorities and conserving energy so as to engage in social activities.

Although the women did not initiate the subject of death and avoided it when the leader mentioned it as a concern, they did talk about the possibility of becoming sicker. The women who lived alone provided hints to one another about safety devices, grocery shopping, home care services, and so forth. All agreed they enjoyed and profited from the meetings.

In addition to the hospital groups other meetings are held in the community and led by community-oriented nurses. These groups provide an opportunity for patients and families to interact outside the hospital setting. People are free to attend these groups at any time but are particularly encouraged to come at the time of initial diagnosis, at recurrence, and when active treatment fails.

Public health and visiting nurses can encourage family members to come to such meetings when the patient is dying. Here they can get support, recognition of the problems they experience, and practical suggestions from others in the same situation. Here too they can be helped to discuss with the patient arrangements regarding his care during this period and whether this should be in hospital or at home.

Problems with Groups

Although we feel that groups are tremendously beneficial to many, it must be recognized that others would prefer to cope on their own or with more individualized attention. This is accepted, and patients are helped to do what is most beneficial for them.

Although groups were initially conceived to save staff time, this has not always been the case. Whereas issues of general concern are raised in the groups, new problems emerge requiring individual attention—primarily because when patients discover staff are willing to help, they are then more likely to discuss personal problems they previously might have hidden. Our belief is that this is essential to the long-range outcome of the illness, and so it is accepted and encouraged.

It has been somewhat surprising to see the tremendous anxiety extremely skilled nurses exhibit at the thought of running such groups. Although these nurses have always dealt well with patients and families on an individual basis, they are panic stricken at the idea of leading a group discussion. This anxiety can be dissipated to some extent through role playing, but for the most part it is resolved as the nurses gain self-confidence in the running of groups with the authors' supervision.

Conclusions

In conclusion it has been our intention to show one method of helping patients and families throughout the course of one life-threatening illness. Rather than concentrating solely on the terminal period, patients and families are given a chance to improve their coping skills throughout the illness. In this way those patients who do become terminal have more support from families and professionals both in the hospital and the community. They are then able to participate in the decisions regarding terminal care and are helped to maintain some independence, dignity, and control during this time.

These weekly meetings are not group therapy but discussion and support groups where patients and families can enter and get help at some of the crucial and transitional periods in living with cancer.

The idea of such groups is not unique to the present authors but can be seen as based on the work of Pratt, who began similar meeting with patients with tuberculosis in 1905. The purpose of his groups was seen as helping patients overcome their discouragement and pessimism, relinquish secondary gains from their illness, and develop increasing self-confidence and self-esteem (Rosenbaum and Berger, 1963). His goals are similar to our own.

Those who have participated as patients have had their questions answered, anxiety relieved, practical help initiated, and hope maintained. Those who have participated as family members are grateful that the terminal period was less stressful than it might otherwise have been.

Acknowledgment

The authors express their appreciation to the staff of Princess Margaret Hospital; the Canadian Cancer Society, Toronto unit; and the staff and patients in the "Coping with Cancer Groups."

References

Lyall, W. A. L., M. L. S. Vachon, and C. P. Nestor. 1973. "Alleviating Stress in the Care of the Dying." Presented at Canadian Psychiatric Association Convention, Vancouver, British Columbia, June.

Rogers, J. and M. L. S. Vachon. 1975. "Nurses Can Help the Bereaved." *Canadian Nurse* 71:61, June.

Rosenbaum, M. and M. Berger. 1963. *Group Psychotherapy and Group Function*. New York: Basic Books.

Vachon, M. L. S. 1972. "Assessing Stress in a Cancer Hospital: A Program of Intervention and Evaluation." Presented at Registered Nurses Association of Ontario, Annual Meeting, Toronto, Ontario, April.

Vachon, M. L. S., A. Formo, K. Freedman, W. A. L. Lyall, J. Rogers, and S. J. J. Freeman. 1976. "Stress Reactions to Bereavement." *Essence* Vol. 1, January.

Vachon, M. L. S. and W. A. L. Lyall. 1976. "Psychiatry and the Patient with Cancer." *Hospital and Community Psychiatry,* June.

⩙⩙⩙ 8

Home Is Not Necessarily "Home"

Steven A. Moss

Home is the sailor, home from the sea,
And the hunter home from the hill.

From the moment of birth, when the infant is expelled from the womb, life is composed of an innumerable series of exits from positions of security until death comes. Each change in life echoes that "birth trauma," as ties are severed and new ones must be knotted, only to be broken again. Each "old" relationship represents calm and peace, while its severance brings on grief, and the establishment of new relationships creates anxiety associated with an unknown future.

I believe that security, peace, roots, are feelings connoted by the word *home,* while insecurity and uprootedness describe the words *diaspora, exile, wandering.* In life, each person yearns for home, not exile. Home, figuratively and literally, is what each person wishes to establish, to return to. And death represents the final return to the state from whence a person came, the final home of complete security and peace. As Rabbi Abraham Heschel (in Riemer, 1974) wrote:

Death may be the beginning of exaltation, an ultimate celebration, a reunion of the divine image with the divine source of being.

Dust returns to dust, while the image, the divine stake in man, is restored to the bundle of life.

Death is not sensed as a defeat but as a summation, a conclusion. . . . The meaning of death is in return, regardless of whether it results in a continuation of individual consciousness or in a merging into a greater whole.

While death as "home" is not yearned for all one's life, when "home" within the context of living cannot be fully achieved, death, that is "to be laid to rest," becomes an alternative over a continued wandering, uprooted existence through life. Such an existence is created by aggravation, anxiety, pain and suffering on physical and emotional levels. It was not difficult for me to understand how death represented a goal of release for a patient I had been visiting who had endured the pain of one operation after another. How often such a patient says, "This is no life." It is not life, for it lacks a sense of security, continuity, self-image, independence, self-worth, and peace—all of which the image of "home" represents. For the sick, and especially for the terminally ill, such a sense of "home" is disturbed, for they are alienated, uprooted, and set apart from their desired state.

Since ancient times, sickness and dying have been viewed as states alien to the social and physical flow of life. In the Bible the leper was cast out of the camp, uprooted from all societal ties. Certain sicknesses, especially those manifested through bodily discharges, were considered to cause a state of uncleanliness in those who suffered from them and in those who cared for the sufferer. Sickness and dying were seen as the results of sin and evil deeds and represented a break between the perpetrator and society, and God. How often the psalmist cried to God to pull him "out of the depths" back into relationship with Him, for in *Sheol,* in death, there is total alienation from God. Such removal from God's presence is similar to exile from home, for in this case God is figuratively "home." As such, repentence, reparation of the broken relationship between man and God, produces a return to God—the place of security.

As long as mankind's knowledge of sickness remained embedded in superstition, fear, and medical ignorance, the sick and dying remained outside the social context physically and emotionally. In Catholicism the priests and nuns, and in Judaism the members of the Holy Brotherhood, the *Chevrah Kadisha,* brought society to the sick and dying. Alienation from society stemmed from fear of physical contagion with the plague, for instance, or from fear of assumed spiritual contagion by dybbukim and spirits. Although, as the middle ages progressed, the dead, who had been excluded from the heart of cities for thousands of years, were intermingled with "the inhabitants of the popular quarters that had been built in the suburbs of the abbeys" (Ariès, 1974). I believe that it would be correct to say that the sick and dying remained either physically, or at least emotionally, apart from the intercourse with daily life. In describing the iconography of the middle ages, Ariès (1974, p. 34) wrote:

The dying man is dying in bed surrounded by his friends and relations. He is in the process of carrying out the rituals which are now familiar to us. But something is happening which disturbs the simplicity of the ceremony and which those present do not see. It is a spectacle reserved for the dying alone and one which he contemplates with a bit of anxiety and a great deal of indifference.

Whereas today one would think that modern medicine's understanding of contagion or disease has helped to alleviate much physical and emotional alienation of the sick and dying, I believe that it really has not. Although the hospital structure, as an institution, is an accepted part of our society, it is still considered a no man's land by many. It is obvious that for these people the hospital is the antithesis of "home," security, independence. As for the nonsick, whose relative or friend is hospitalized, the institution remains alien territory, tinged with fear and anxiety. Many people refuse to visit either a hospital or a cemetery. Some of these, I believe, have a superstitious fear of the unknown, as well as of contagion by the unwanted. I was appalled when a modern, middle-aged person asked me whether or not cancer was contagious. The answer would influence his visiting his dying friend.

Much in recent literature has been written about this alienation of the sick and dying. For many, for most, the hospital and surely the nursing home or health-related facility are not "home." As Ariès (1974, pp. 88–89) wrote:

Death in the hospital is no longer the occasion of a ritual ceremony, over which the dying presides amidst his assembled relatives and friends. Death is a technical phenomenon obtained by a cessation of care, a cessation determined in a more or less avowed way by a decision of the doctor and the hospital team. Indeed, in the majority of cases the dying person has already lost consciousness. . . . Today the initiative has passed from the family, as much an outsider as the dying person, to the doctor and the hospital team. They are the masters of death. . . .

But even these "masters of death" stay away from the patient. How often the surgeon ceases seeing a patient, or visits him only sporadically and briefly, because now that patient has become terminal! How often the nurse establishes her priorities on the basis of which patients are dying, and therefore in need of extended emotional more than physical nursing, and focuses her efforts on those patients who will get well, more in need of physical nursing, with its more positive results. During my chaplaincy visits I am faced frequently by the question, "Why doesn't anyone stop in to see me?" If I were to answer, "because you are dying," I would probably be right.

The feeling of alienation is further enhanced by family or friends, who, out of guilt, fear of open communication, or even anticipatory grief, withdraw from the dying patient. It would seem, then, that this task of establishing relationships, creating an atmosphere of "home," is left primarily to the nonmedical staffs. But how much can they do, and how many of them are not always successful either, because of their own difficulties of working with the dying, although within their chosen professions they must be brought into contact with them?

Given this meaning of the word *home,* and how it connotes warmth, fulfilled and genuine relationships, security, life with meaning, being a person, I can understand why so many patients want very badly to go home. Home is, however, a quality as much as a place, and so I have met those who would rather be in a hospital setting than at home, because their homes are not really "home."

Ideally, a dying patient's home should have the qualities of which I have written. To ensure the presence of these qualities is certainly no easy task. But if home care of the living patient who is dying is to be real "home" care, at least these qualities ought to be present to some degree. How can they be achieved?

I would answer that it is necessary to treat the dying patient as a person, that is, another being with a whole range of needs, desires, and hopes, despite a limited life expectancy. All too often, even when the patient is home, the family continues the same nonperson, alienating treatment of the patient as they did when in the hospital. The family, as well as outsiders coming in, withdraw from "real" relationships with the dying because they fail to understand that a dying person still has the need for meaningful tasks, goals, and so forth; they fear that they will be hurt if the relationship is too involved when death occurs (therefore anticipatory grief comes into being); and they really do not know what to do with the dying, for they assume that such deeds can have no relationship with what one does with and for the living.

These three reasons for withdrawal from the dying, along with others, cause the dying to experience home as "not home," to experience being treated as nonpersons. As has been written of the hospital (Kutscher and Goldberg, 1973), so too can it be applied to a home that is not "home":

The dying usually finds himself being abandoned as his condition deteriorates; the living have already "written him off." He becomes the central figure in a great "conspiracy of silence"—forbidden to voice his fears and lied to concerning his condition and progress.

The process of home care of the dying is to establish the qualities of "home" life. As much as possible, life at home should continue as previously. Relationships and roles should remain constant. No person should become a saint overnight unless such a metamorphosis is genuinely felt (i.e., to relieve future guilt). I have found in my chaplaincy work that the dying do not want to be burdens on others, and one way that can be felt is if, all of a sudden, old family patterns and schedules are changed. The dying want life to go on as usual. They usually want the children to remain in school and the husband to continue working. For the lives of others to change is for others to consider the dying, not as a person, but as an object, an invalid, and a burdensome one at that. Home, then, would represent insecurity, guilt, and changed relationships.

Within physical limitations, the dying can still carry on activities as before, so as to be fulfilled intellectually, emotionally, spiritually, and existentially. It might mean that office work needs to be brought home, although as much as possible a dying person with an office job should be allowed to spend some time in those important and fulfilling surroundings; or a volunteer group of which the dying person is a member,.from the synagogue or church, can come to the house. No one can assume that a dying person no longer has desire or drive to accomplish. If limitations are too great to continue what was done in the past, meaningful new tasks can be created—from study to painting or creative writing (dictation can be a substitute for writing). A person is one who has meaning in life. Home is where one can freely find and express meaning. I believe that the dying person should not be exempt from either. As Frankl (1967) wrote:

It is precisely when facing such a fate, when being confronted with a hopeless situation, that man is given a last opportunity to fulfill a meaning—to realize even the highest value, to fulfill even the deepest meaning—and that is the meaning of suffering. . . . Life's transitoriness does not in the least detract from its meaningfulness.

It is my intention here that the continuance of prior relationships and roles in the family and the furtherance of life-verifying tasks for the dying will create home as "home." Once these patterns of behavior can be achieved on some level, I believe that the living will further intensify the treatment of the dying person, for they will see that the dying person *is* still a person and not a new subspecies of human being to be treated differently, with fear and trembling. The living will see that, when relationships with the dying, and especially those who are loved ones, are fulfilled through intense, meaning-verifying relationships until the very end, then hurt from guilt or frustration will be minimized when death occurs. The sting of death would be somewhat eased because of the realization that *all* was done to continue to sustain meaning in the face of death. Something was done by the loved one who treated the dying as a person, making home a "home," until the end.

These, then, are a few of my suggestions for making the home of the dying to be truly like "home." And for those who cannot go home but are in honest need of a health-related facility, nursing home, or chronic and terminal facility, it is my idealistic hope that some day such facilities will have the type of staff and environment that can make such an institution like a "home," whereby life-verifying goals, tasks, and relationships can be confirmed until death comes. Surely, the already established hospices in this country and abroad are a step in this direction.

I have written this analysis of the treatment of the dying, and a few suggestions to better this treatment, in the hope that home care of the dying can be real "home" care, whether at home or in an institution. Home is a quality, not just a place. While dying must be a lonely experience, it need not be an alienated, depersonalized one. To combat such a feeling is to establish the quality of "home" wherever the dying live.

References

Ariès, P. 1974. *Western Attitudes Toward Death: From the Middle Ages to the Present*. Baltimore: Johns Hopkins University Press, p. 18.

Frankl, V. 1967. *Psychotherapy and Existentialism*. New York: Simon and Schuster, pp. 14–15.

Kutscher, A. H. and M. Goldberg, eds. 1973. *Caring for the Dying Patient and His Family* New York: Health Sciences Publishing Corp., p. 16.

Riemer, J., ed. *Jewish Reflections on Death*. New York: Schocken Books.

For Further Reading
Riemer, J. 1974. Jewish Reflections on Death. New York: Schocken Books, pp. 64–65.

Family Involvement with the Dying Patient

Althea Dean and Abraham Lurie

An acute-care hospital is prepared to provide a battery of sophisticated medicated services to patients both on an inpatient and an outpatient basis. For many seriously ill patients, involvement with such a hospital continues over a period of years and ranges through surgical procedures, chemotherapy, radiation therapy, and supportive followup therapy in the clinic or from the affiliated private physician. Other patients may have had only a single and relatively brief contact with the hospital, the remainder of their medical care being furnished in their physician's office. Nevertheless, the hospital is usually the primary resource, the haven, for patients combating fatal diseases. When nothing more can be done for them medically, these patients, now dying, are cared for in a terminal facility, a nursing home, or their own home. Whereas hospital inpatient beds are devoted to other patients who can still benefit from life-saving procedures, techniques, and devices, we are concerned with the home-based patient who is expected to remain at home until death.

Administratively, an acute-care hospital is set up so that patients with incurable diseases and grave prognoses can be identified at the

84

time of their entry into the system. Social work intervention at this point varies from actual crisis intervention to a more sustained information-giving approach, depending on the stage of the disease and the ability of the patient and family to cope with what is happening to them at that time. No patient should, however, leave the hospital without knowing that social work services are available to patient and family when and if needed.

Many adjustments need to be made by patient and family, not only to the disease and its prognosis, but also to the realities that intrude and must be faced. Few newly diagnosed patients or families are familiar with the technicalities they will soon be facing in terms of such basics as insurance coverage; resources for housekeeping, baby sitting, or transportation assistance; and negotiating the tradeoffs necessary to ensure the maximum income through retirement or disability or pension benefits. These are the least emotionally threatening areas and are usually the most pressing. The social worker often begins by dealing with these, not only out of necessity but also because it is sometimes easier during this stage for the patient and his family to deal with concrete needs and planning than it is to allow themselves to feel the total impact of what is happening to them. The sudden onrush of huge medical, hospital, and doctor bills overwhelms the average person. Many react by depleting savings, cashing in insurance policies, and taking out loans with little thought of how they will be repaid, in a form of bargaining—"spend enough and you will be cured." It is common to see families spending money they can ill afford for private-duty nurses, specialized equipment, and similar services when all that is actually needed is help with meal preparation and supportive companionship. The social worker has a direct role in channeling the family's resources and should have considerable expertise in the ins and outs of managing an illness from the nonmedical point of view. The patient and family must be helped to see what their options are and what the consequences of various concrete approaches are and must be firmly supported in conserving energies and finances for when they may be more urgently needed.

There are appropriate community resources to which the social worker can direct the family suddenly facing a fatal illness and experiencing hard-core needs they have not known before. A family emotionally overburdened in coping with long-drawn-out terminal illness and apparently unsophisticated about community resources may not be aware that for them the most beneficial service from the community might be day camp for the young child in the family or tickets to the ballgame for the teenager in the family. There are small foundations and funds that can be tapped for these purposes in the same way that larger groups are prepared to give assistance with the more readily identifiable needs, such as homemaker service equipment.

It is important to know the individual dynamics in each patient and family group and to understand that they are not necessarily manifested simultaneously or compatibly by both patient and family. The patient may be seething with anger and rage at his diagnosis and prognosis, while family members are still denying their reality. Nor is it unusual to find a despairing and depressed patient the members of whose family are so overwhelmed with their own anger that they can be of little comfort and help to the patient. Social work intervention is directed at helping resolve the individual and interpersonal conflicts and at enabling patient and family to move toward better adaptation.

Although medical care from a large medical center or acute-care hospital is probably vastly superior to what was rendered in the "good old days" by the "family doctor," there is less of a sense of continuity as the medical treatment progresses. Patients are passed from the internist to the surgeons to the oncologist to the radiologist and to the other medical and nonmedical specialists. It is often not clear who is actually the managing physician. Continuity is vital, and it is a characteristic of the constant support and availability of the social worker familiar since the first hospitalization.

Depending on their own supports, their coping patterns, and the other psychosocial factors that influence the impact of the illness and of the impending death, patients and families make differential use of the service offered by social workers. The elderly widow, aware that she is dying from cancer and concerned about her emotionally disturbed daughter's ability to care for her grandchild, can make good use of her relationship with the social worker. This patient has someone with whom she can talk openly about her unwillingness to die until the granddaughter's future is more safely assured, her sense of failure at her daughter's inability to function adequately as a mother, and her anger at, and envy of, those who are still young and healthy. With advice from the social worker she can begin to plan for the child and become involved with a community agency that will continue as a resource even after her death.

It has been our experience that, before much else can be accomplished, the anger of both patient and family must be recognized, supported, and ventilated. Society permits, although with some discomfort, the dying patient to be angry—to ask, "Why me?" and to exhibit some regressive and primitive behavior. He cannot be too strongly criticized. At the same time he is encouraged to "cheer up," while the denial of those around him is foisted upon him. He is told by caring friends and relatives that he is "looking better" and will soon be well. In the same manner the wife (or husband or parent) is applauded for her faithfulness, her tireless attention to the patient, and her "appropriate" concern and grief. Any expression of anger or fear by the family member at his or her own situation; any sign of frustration over the consequences to be anticipated at the loss of income or having to abandon vacation or travel plans brings instant disapproval.

As early as possible, the social worker tries to help the family members and the patient ventilate these negative feelings and support those feelings where valid. Only then can the patient or family move ahead in dealing with the impending loss. A 45-year-old narcissistic woman, whose husband was dying at home, was actually neglecting his care, appeared indifferent to his pain, and had alienated family, friends, and the physician by her complaints of her own suffering. Social work intervention at this point resulted in the wife's ready verbalization of her rage that she would soon have to give up her nice apartment, that their long-planned vacation to Las Vegas for their twenty-fifth anniversary would never take place, that her handsome husband was no longer handsome, and that she would belong nowhere at all in this "couple's society" and would be too old to compete with younger women. She was so involved with her own losses that she had no energy for anything else, and those around her would not tolerate her verbalization of "selfish" needs "at a time like this." Once these feelings were explored and sorted out and her materialistic losses put in better perspective, the wife was able to be more supportive to the patient and ultimately to let him know the full depth of her caring. Close family members have a stake in the patient's well-being and can be helped to extend therapeutic support.

Another patient, dying of leukemia, could not deal with his anger and became uncharacteristically caustic and cruel to his wife, while presenting his usual and gracious demeanor to everyone else. The social worker's role was to connect this man with his anger, channelize it appropriately, and direct it to the right source. Then he could share with his wife their mutual sense of grief at the losses both were facing. When anger is appropriately expressed and channeled, supports emerge from many sources—friends, family, medical people, and others with whom relationships have developed.

As the illness progresses, psychosocial needs of the patient and family vary, and the supportive role of the social worker may become more or less intensive, ranging from regularly scheduled to a more intuitive, "as needed," contact. Often the social work emphasis may shift from the parents to the child or children, and the expectation that they will need fairly intensive support or psychotherapy. Again this depends on the individual circumstances, but it is usual to have specialized help available on behalf of the child who is losing a parent. Whereas we meet some of the patients' and families' needs from the hospital-based social work department, since their medical needs are being met or monitored from the hospital, resources for projected continuing needs of a surviving child are more likely to be sought from the nonmedical community—a child guidance agency, community youth group, or other social agency particularly oriented to the needs of youngsters.

There are distressing gaps in service for the dying patient and his family. Only the relatively affluent can afford both the bare necessities and the amenities. The very poor and the low-income groups, while covered in some ways by public funds, must often find a way to pay for costly supplies, dressings, and nonprescription items not covered by state or federal medical programs. But the most conspicuous and compelling need is for inpatient care of the terminally ill whose care can no longer be managed at home and whose medical needs do not warrant acute hospital care. This might include those whose family members no longer have the physical stamina to turn, lift, and otherwise care for the patient. Of most concern to us, however, are those patients whose intractable pain cannot be managed at home. Such pain requires the daily, often hourly, attention and sophisticated knowledge of a physician. The average nursing home is not a viable alternative to inpatient hospital care under these circumstances. Within a 50-mile radius of the hospital with which the authors are connected there are two facilities for terminal care. Both of these are accessible to the families of patients from this area only by automobile and fail, therefore, to meet an important criterion: that the patient have his family with him. It confirms for many that one must be "sent away" to die.

Social workers are beginning to share with each other their experience, knowledge, and compelling goal for better care of dying patients. Social workers have considerable expertise in establishing certain psychosocial criteria for adequate health care; these should be combined with those of other disciplines to meet patient needs. The terminal care facility or hospice can be implemented on the community level in a tentative way by using existing nursing homes or similar facilities and staffing one wing or one floor with adequate and appropriate personnel. This could and should be the joint project of several community-based hospitals that serve a common geographic area. Social workers must continue to document these needs and join with physicians, nurses, administrators, clergy, and community groups in pressing for the most feasible, appropriate, and direct solutions readily available.

≈≈≈ 10

"He's a Sick Man—
He Belongs in the Hospital"

Naomi Bluestone

"I heard old Mrs. Rubin is bringing her Joe home from the hospital on Tuesday."

"What, him in his condition?"

"Well, all I know is she said they were calling the ambulance for Tuesday morning."

"What's the matter with those people sending him out! Why he's a dying man if ever I saw one. Did you see the way he looked?"

"Not this time. But I saw him the last time they took him in and he looked like death warmed over *then,* all skin and bones and that glassy look. I tell you the truth, I don't know how she's going to be able to take it, him being around all the time."

"Well, I guess you're right. They oughtta be ashamed, letting him out in his condition. That poor woman wouldn't even be able to lift him, and who's to help her?"

"I heard her daughter, the one that lives upstairs, she's working half-time for a while."

"That's no solution. She's got her own life to lead, and her kids need her.

90

They're at the age. Do you think maybe they ought to put him in a nursing home? I heard he can't even walk to the toilet any more."

"What do you want, she should feel guilty after all these years? Look, how much longer can he last? And where is he going to go? From what I hear, I wouldn't put a dog in one of those places. They take worse care of you than they do in a hospital. And who's paying for all of this? So long he was in the hospital, I bet they don't have a penny left. That Medicare is a gyp."

"Oh, she's not on Medicare, they got some money."

"Not Medicaid, Medicare."

"Well, whatever it is, by the time she'll get through with the nurses and the social workers and the this and the that, she'll be cleaned out good, Medicare or no Medicare. I don't think she's doing right by him. She should have left him in the hospital."

"And maybe she didn't have a choice? You know those doctors. The minute they're through with you, they want to get you out. They don't care what happens to you. She's gonna have her hands full. That poor soul, you mark my words, she's gonna have her hands full."

"Maybe you should tell her?"

"What should I tell her? Is it *my* business I should tell her? I'll bring her a cake, what else can I do?"

"You're right. But you know what I think?"

"What?"

"I think he's a sick man. He belongs in the hospital!"

The well-defined period preceding marriage is known to us as the courtship or engagement, and we have a variety of colloquial terms to describe the advent of less formal liaisons. But to the best of my knowledge we have no term at all to designate the period, years later, in which a couple knowingly await the termination of the marriage through the death of one of the partners. The great lexicographers who have given us such scientific and inventive terms as "neoplasm" (new growth) and "pleonasm" (a redundancy) have never seen fit to legitimate this very real waiting period with a noun of its own. Nevertheless, it is a most crucial period, and commonly the participants prefer to spend it in familiar surroundings, at home rather than in the hospital. But how can this longing for home be reconciled with

"He's a sick man; he belongs in a hospital," an equally impelling modern urban ethic? Often it cannot, and the conflict rages between these two poles from the first day the sick person is centrifuged into the hospital until the day he or she departs the world.

I am concerned here with the tug of war between home and hospital, in which the grass always seems greener where the patient is not, and the whispers of the neighbors provide as much impetus for admission and discharge as the counsels of the professionals. It is important because the ambivalence the dipolarization produces creates tremendous pressures on medical care and takes an exhausting toll of the available physical and emotional stamina of families.

Perhaps I can begin by examining some of the common feelings and thought processes surrounding the transfer of persons such as Mr. Rubin (who is fictitious, as are his wife and the two neighbors so anxious to mind her business for her).

It commonly occurs that the moment a seriously ill man enters the hospital, his wife cannot wait to get him home. Her prayers are a verbal talisman: "Please Lord, just let me get him home. I can handle anything as long as I have him home. Please let him come home again and I'll never ask you for anything else again as long as I live." (Spouses bargain, too!) But when the ambulance comes for the ride home, her heart fails. In panic she relives each of her husband's crises and asks herself if she could have handled them at home. She scrutinizes his every expression and gesture to see if a relapse is imminent. She forgets the bad nursing experiences and remembers only the good ones. Acutely aware that support is being withdrawn, she tells herself that, if anything happens, she can always bring him back. Yet she also knows that if she *does* have to bring him back one more time, they'll have to make up a bed for *her*, too.

Much has been written about the excitement and drama of the ambulance ride *to* the hospital, sirens screaming, traffic melting, but for our purposes, it is the trip home again that is most symbolic. It represents a dramatic weaning on wheels, a sharp separation from a provident institution that traditionally demands total helplessness and submission until the very instant of discharge and then, as George S. Kaufman put it so well, "kicks baby's rosy bottom out into the snow." When the ambulance deposits her and roars off, she is remarkably alone.

Now, what does she find? She finds that the familiar home she has lived in for so long suddenly seems strange and queer. The big, hulking man who used to come bounding up the stairs two at a time now must be lifted like a baby. The heavy work that she used to nag him to do accumulates, while she exhausts herself handwashing pajamas. Every service he requires is punctuated by the terror that it will not be done properly. Habits, adjustments, relationships of a lifetime are shifted. Let me present just one small example. If she sleeps in the same bedroom with him, as she has for 40 years, she is awake all night, tense each time he turns. But if she sleeps on the sofa bed in the guest room, she worries that she will not hear him if he should call. Furthermore, she sees it as a rejection, a sign of defeat, a tangible evidence of the change in their relationship, and worst of all, a forerunner of the longer separation to come. So, she catnaps during the day, chronically tired.

Although she is brave, she may occasionally need to break down, but she cannot even find a place to do that. In the hospital, she could take a walk around the block if she wanted a good cry, but now where can she go? To the kitchen? To put her head in the oven? It won't do . . . her puffy eyes will betray her. The relief at having him home is tempered with the reality problems known so well by all, and as time wears on, the hints of neighbors and the suggestions of family urge her to "consider alternatives." There are few. Like a serpent tempting Eve, the thought that has come full circle keep recurring: "He's a sick man. He belongs in the hospital!" And she is primed for the ambulance to come again at the first crisis.

So now we come to the essence. *Where did that idea come from?* Is it true? Is it a twentieth-century old wives' tale? Does it represent an understandable dumping syndrome developed by families in response to stress on the home front? Or is it an artificial situation, contrived and promulgated by the profession itself, that has inflated expectations and unfairly enticed careworn people who have actually exhausted the specialized services of the hospital? Is it a siren song from the hospital itself, which readmits patients the way mechanics readmit cars, on the basis of a rattle, a groan, or a hysterical driver? Or is it a product of the legal, financial, insurance, and malpractice interests, which ensure readmissions on the same principles by which general practitioners now order x-rays of small bones? To what extent can we recognize and reverse an inappropriate custom that demands automatic hospitalization for the critically ill patient who threatens everyone with his terrible needs and his tangible dying?

The answers to these questions must unfortunately be conjectural, but certain facts are not. Despite all our knowledge about the needs of terminally ill patients, and the acceptability of hospices established to provide the services they require, there are still few alternatives. In America, hospices are token, and nursing homes routinely induce senile marasmus. Home care programs are bleak and pinched, anemic and attenuated. In hospitals, admitting residents resent bed occupancy by terminally ill persons the way the Parisiens smoldered under occupation of their homes by the Germans. Indeed the medical profession, which has produced more specialties than the marrow yields corpuscles, will go only to the brink and no farther; surely the only reason it has failed to establish board certification in "clinical thanatology" (as a subspecialty of internal medicine) is that it does not consider death to come within its purview at all. (Just imagine the bizarre questions the qualifying examination might require: "List the 96 causes of death.")

In the last analysis, most families are forced to play "home–nursing home–hospital hopscotch," with the patient as puck. No matter what our opinions may be regarding the priorities that have determined this country's well-studied policy of "semi-intensive abandonment," to rail against them today would be but one more example of the propensity of caring persons to ruminate and decompress fruitlessly among themselves in lieu of purposeful action. What, instead, can we do to ease the burden of the Mrs. Rubins of this world? What, realistically, can we offer them? One thing we can do is teach our patients and their families exactly what a hospital can and cannot do. A realistic understanding on the consumer level of the purpose, environment, ambiance, staffing, equipment, advantages, and drawbacks of each of the health services institutions would enable families to be more realistic when the need for an escape begins to manifest, and pressure for relief and change starts to mount. The lack of community between families of expiring persons prevents dissemination of this hard-won knowledge. Too often it is learned through trial and error, after repeated admissions have failed to meet expectations.

I can think of no advantage to forcing a sick and wretched individual to discover afresh that the hospital is *not* a place to get a rest, *not* a place in which he can be taken care of, *not* a place in which he will be protected and safe, but rather a maddening environment, which frequently breeds rage, resentment, frustration, self-pitying outrage, unbridled fury, terror, helplessness, powerlessness, and aggravation. If you do not believe that, lie in a hospital bed some day and watch a dietary aide throw a dinner tray down on your bedside table, just out of reach. Ring for the nurse to come and move it 6 inches closer to your nose, so that you can manipulate it with your unparalyzed hand. Then wait 57 minutes, as it grows ice cold in front of your eyes.

Another helpful movement would be to try to come to grips with the great American hospital transference. I believe there is a real "institutional neurosis" in this country, in which patients, whose needs for consolation are unmet by impersonal physicians, seek care and nurturing from the large, concrete hospital, which holds at least the promise of more receptivity. Persons having difficulty with the inexorability of disease are particularly susceptible to the temptation to denigrate a physician's pronouncements and push on to the Delphic installation with the ICU. Fifty years ago the great city hospitals were places where people were taken, kicking and screaming, to die, because little could be done for them. Now the doors of these same institutions are being kicked down for the same purpose—after *everything* has been done.

Families should be encouraged to have some faith in their own ability to provide adequate care for a patient with intensive nursing needs, given proper support and training. The expropriation of health services by the white army should be reversed. At a time when nursing services have become so downgraded that relatively untrained and unskilled persons now provide most basic personal services in institutions, it is hard to believe that families still think that a "nurse" can provide better service than love and willing hands. The utter passivity and ignorance of these families in the face of so-called professionals is a most repellent paradox. I recall, when working on a geriatric ward of a state hospital, how meekly families would permit themselves to be shooed away from the bedside, so that a totally uncaring, heavy-handed stevedore in a dirty white cap could haul their wife and mother around like an old carton being chased by a washrag.

Perhaps several more points should be emphasized. We should not shy away from increasing the in-community experience of families with terminally ill relatives, as long as an institution is truly not needed. Isolation and estrangement tend to increase the push toward hospitalization, and the presence of peer relationships in the community can be a great buttress. Furthermore, we need greater emphasis on control of pain and discomfort at home. Traditional barriers against the use of certain drugs, for example, need investigation under the special circumstances raised by patients who will not recover.

Lastly, the various components of the "grass is greener" syndrome should be studied further, if only because the pressure of neighbors and friends in times of great stress is a tremendous impetus for unnecessary hospitalization. "He's a sick man. He belongs in a hospital" is an ethic deriving from an unseemly dependence on an imperfect system by a confused family. Its most consistent characteristic is the ease with which it reverses itself, and the ambivalence it perpetuates, indicators of a duality we would do well to understand.

"Joe's had those choking spells for three weeks, why did she fall apart like that?"

"I don't know, but when you're all alone in the middle of the night like that, what else was she going to do?"

"Well, I just can't see taking him back to the hospital when you and I both know there isn't a thing they can do for him. When you're that sick sometimes you should stay out of the hospital."

"Do you think it was because the daughter had to go back to work? I know that's been a worry on her."

"So what's so terrible? You never heard of home care? Dora had her brother-in-law on home care for years. The minute he went back into the hospital, he got an infection and started going down again."

"Look, *I* never said it was such a good idea, her taking him to the hospital. Don't I know what hospitals are like? All night he could lie and call, and no one would answer his bell, believe me!"

"You're close to her . . . maybe you should tell her?"

"I did tell her. 'Listen' I said, 'what are you doing? Take my advice! He's a sick man. He doesn't belong in a hospital!' "

"So what did she say?"

"Nothing! What could she say!"

⚜⚜⚜ 11

In Favor of House Calls

Charles Adsit

As a physician, Vladimir Owens was too good to be true—he made house calls, and this aroused his patients' suspicions. . . . detectives arrested him for not being the physician he pretended to be.

Informed of the case, the American Medical Association was taken aback. "House calls," an association spokesman said, "are extremely inefficient" (New York Times, Dec. 13, 1974).

There are other hazards to house calls. For instance, in New York City, the $95-a-throw tow-away program. In some slightly more remote areas, just outside New York's city limits, there are no doubt dangers of plane crashes, blizzards, rattlesnakes, and wolf packs. But home care is not possible without the house call.

In whose view is the house call "extremely inefficient"? Certainly not that of the patient or his family, and do we all not give quick lip service to stating that it is the patient who matters and whose care is paramount? Is this negative attitude not a transparent copout on the part of the professed physician?

Consider the mental state of the family who knows that the attending physician does not make house calls. Surely it must appear that "I'll take care of you as long as it is convenient, and you can come to my office or to the hospital; if things get tough and you cannot leave your bed, you will have to get someone else to take care of you''—a secondary physician, only secondarily interested, who resents not being chosen in the first place. Consider the panic that strikes if these facts come out for the first time in a crisis.

Is a house call inefficient, even from the point of view of the physician? One cannot expect to understand a full picture by viewing only a fragment. To see a patient in one's office or in the isolation of a hospital room is to view only a fragment—a single cell separated from its basic tissue. In no time at all it is possible on a house call to get considerable insight into both physical and psychological areas invisible in any other setting and yet totally basic and essential for sympathetic understanding. Tiresome questions need not be asked or answered; one has but to observe.

The mere fact of the presence of the physician in the home provides comfort and relative peace of mind for both family and patient; tensions relax, pain is eased. Even in a hopeless situation something is being done to help. If things get worse, my doctor will come again to see me. Certainly if a choice had to be made, the dying patient would trade all the computerized ivory towers in the world for a human being willing to help in every way possible.

The physician does benefit from this relationship. Often the mechanical problems of patient care are more difficult for the seriously sick than the medical management. These problems can best be understood *in situ;* not uncommonly, small changes and adjustments can greatly improve patient comfort. A check of the medicine cabinet may be enough to identify high-sodium items being ingested but not viewed as medication by the patient, explaining edema states that would otherwise require additional drugs for relief. A view of the bookshelves will give insight into hobbies, literary interests, and past life-style of the family, providing multiple subjects for diversionary conversation. Family photographs give a happier view of days when things were better; the past provides many clues to the present. In short, the patient's home is a rich mine of information available from no other source.

But this source is available not only to the internist or general practitioner. The hospital-based specialist should see to it that he visits this wellspring frequently; it will open up to him a whole new and more rewarding world of warm, personal contact he can obtain in no other way in the practice of medicine; in fact this is what the practice of medicine is all about. One can go only so far in the doctor-patient relationship in an office or hospital. This applies to each specialist—psychiatrist, surgeon, neurologist, radiotherapist, whatever. The home visit provides an added dimension; theory becomes reality. The patient feels that, no matter how ill he becomes, he will not be rejected and abandoned, and the physician will be amply rewarded for his investment of time and inconvenience.

Surely the dying patient deserves this extra effort, and most certainly the busiest of specialists could schedule one such patient visit a week. Even if the patient himself becomes too ill to get the most out of the house call, the physician is helping the family build a stronger bridge over their grief. Other members of the concerned team—nurse, homemaker, social worker, minister, family friends, and neighbors—all will be equally aided in carrying out this difficult joint endeavor, the support and gentle rescue of the patient as he is guided with all possible skill past the lonely and terrifying aspects of dying. The image of medicine itself will benefit. For once no one loses. House calls should be made.

⚘⚘⚘ 12

The Patient's Home Is His Castle

Anne Gayner

I am suddenly back in time ruminating over events that were so devastating that I can't help but marvel at the human being's capacity to endure the unendurable. I talk not only of the dying; I talk of those who must go on living.

My husband died four years ago. Just being able to use the word *died* instead of the euphemisms with which I had protected myself shows me how much I have grown in these most difficult years. Trying to explain my reactions and overreactions to myself has given me an insight that only those who have traveled this desolate route can recognize. This recognition obliges me to share with others the emotional needs of the dying and the bereaved. The greatest memorial I can give my husband is to tell it like it was, like it is, and like it should be.

This paper is based on vignettes and on a diary written down in shorthand, in guarded privacy, during the time he was ill and after he died. Upon reflection I know that the act of recording events and thoughts helped me keep my sanity at a time when I was compelled, through circumstances, to lead the life of a self-imposed ''schizophrenic.'' It is incomprehensible to me now, that the very people—doctors, family, nurses, and clergy—who could have eased our burden perpetuated instead a denial that resulted in unresolved grief and delayed acceptance. What I did not know then was that they could not ease it, because they did not know how to handle their own emotions and attitudes toward death. Everybody was protecting everybody else, and therein lies the lie.

When it was over, I knew that there had to be a better way to die and to live. I am grateful that I had the courage of my convictions to follow through and find some answers in the face of "the chapter is closed," "it is morbid to talk of death," "life goes on." These very clichés had led me into the trap of denial, and I was not about to let this happen again if I was to lead a meaningful life.

Not until six months after Henry's surgery was I told that the leiomyoscarcoma had metastasized to his liver and that the doctor had thought he would never leave the hospital. How could I have been so naive as to believe that he would be well! Yes, it was fortuitous to have had this elective surgery for the polyp in his colon (which indeed was benign as predicted), for it disclosed the cancer on his jejunum that was not visible on x-ray. "Oh sure," was the reply to my question, "he can live another 30 years that way, can't he?" I was elated at the false prognosis and walked on air doubly enjoying every minute in my ignorance of the future. I felt lucky that we had caught it in time.

Why should he have been told that it was malignant? Both of his parents had died of cancer, and his father had tried to commit suicide. Anyway, he was going to make a complete recovery, and so it would serve no purpose to alarm him. When the bomb was dropped six months later, in my own doctor's office as he told me the truth, I had to "control myself" because my husband was parking the car, and I expected to find him in the waiting room. This doctor, who was a true friend, told me what we should have known from the beginning. For three and a half years I had to learn to live with death, trying to cram as much of life as possible into our numbered days together.

I followed the not unique route of tracking down surgeons, doctors, and clergy, looking for advice, answers, and miracles, all while having to "keep a stiff upper lip." When my husband came home humming (that's how I always knew he was at the door), I assured myself that it was better for him "not to know" and in secret took my private tranquilizers. There is no turning back. The deceit, deception, and intrigue between each and among family, friends, and doctors cannot be described or believed. At a time when we had the biggest problem of our lives to share, I was forced to smile and deny.

One does not go through three and one-half years of watching her husband die of terminal cancer and four years of widowhood without physical and psychological scarring. But in the healing of those scars there are some positive aspects. There is the ability to emphathize with those who have and will "walk in my moccasins." While they are not dainty, they are sturdy from having weathered many bumpy roads.

I had contact with many doctors. Not all of them had the same philosophy. Whereas there are no clear-cut rules for death and dying, and the doctors take their cues from the patient, we can influence those cues and come to believe the unbelievable. I wrote a retrospective note that I never had the courage to mail:

Dear Doctors:
This story needs no introduction. You all knew Henry and, unfortunately, haven't been able to escape me. I know that I have been difficult to understand and have driven more than one person up the proverbial wall (always begging for blood), but I must get the following off my heavy chest and overactive mind. Contrary to popular opinion, I have not been wallowing in the depths of widowhood but have been actively engaged in the grieving process, which has been harder than any work one will ever be called on to do. In order to achieve this end and come to grips with the "whys" of living, one must honestly reveal rather than conceal the "wise" of dying. It is for this reason that I find it necessary and important to share some of the insights that come from thinking through.

Perhaps it is in the form of an apology for listening to your words but not absorbing meanings behind them. Perhaps it is because I felt so self-conscious about crying out for help when my distress signals took up so much of your valuable time. But, you see, Henry and I didn't have that much time, and frustration and helplessness alter behavior. Everytime I think my own end might be near (and none of us has any contracts), I feel that I can't leave without giving this feedback. I've drawn up my will, I've donated my eyes, but my life won't be in order until I've made a contribution to the dying and bereaved who will come after me. That's more important than any antiques I will ever leave. I'll probably wheeze along until I'm 100, but, just in case, I'd better get it down on paper.

I realize now that I am not just half of Henry but all of me. It has not been easy to attain this growth. It has come at the expense of much fight and flight adrenalin and resultant physical destruction. If ever anyone needs an example of what repressed rage in the face of hopelessness can do, I am a willing guinea pig. My husband was the only one who counted, and I see now that this was not fair—not fair to him and not fair to myself. How I wanted to cry in his arms and be comforted. How I wanted to unburden myself to my children, only to be held back by a strong sense of "why make them miserable too." The fact of the matter is we had to be miserable because something so devastating was happening to each one of us. We were losing a beautiful person—husband, father, and son. My own father died five weeks before my husband. I wanted to cry in his arms too and ask this biblical scholar, "Where is God? What is happening to us?" But I was protecting him too. That is, I thought I was.

Yes, I felt cheated and defeated and led a self-imposed double life, screaming on the inside and facade-like on the outside. Keeping up pretenses is not only intolerable and out of character but also very destructive psychologically. I consumed enormous amounts of medication both for physical pain (fractured leg) and mental anguish, all of which clouded the issues that had to be faced in order to achieve healthy resolution.

This was done on the assumption that it was better for the patient. But was it really? Perhaps at the beginning it was, but then when it becomes impossible, and eye-avoiding lies lead to lack of communication, there is no turning back, and what should be a meaningful parting of life becomes a terrifying game. When one is going through a period of reconstruction, there must be truth, and the truth, I have found through bitter experience, is not nearly as awesome as the lies to evade it. I deluded myself in primitive thinking and expended energy trying to deny and convince Henry to deny, when that energy should have been expended toward acceptance of the inevitable.

I know lots of things now that I didn't know or didn't want to know then. I learned not only from traveling this desolate route but also from talking to others who had made this same journey. It is little comfort to know that my reactions and overreactions were not unique but instead were responses to extreme denial and an unwillingness to accept reality. It is wrong to usurp someone's right to know what is happening to him. It is also an enormous responsibility to the usurper. When a couple has shared all of the joys and problems that come with living together for 31 years and then can't share the biggest problem of all, it is unjust, unfair, and unreal. Just getting

Henry to go to the doctor resulted in tension. I had to scheme and plan and urge and lie.

There was an air of intrigue where there should have been deep communication that people only know when they have cried in each other's arms. It is a catharsis for both souls who have learned to care so much for the needs of each other. This we did when our true emotions spilled over, but then I felt guilty about our being depressed and again assumed the role of "everything will be all right." Now I see the ludicrousness of the situation. Why shouldn't we have been depressed? We were losing each other. I say "we" because as I did things I asked myself "What is better for Henry?" It should have been, "What is better for us?" Emotions and feelings need venting. When the escape valve is sealed, the explosion must occur. It is a law of physics and a law of life, the basis for all human relationships. He and I were part of the same life-threatened situation.

I have been applauded and commended for the "amazing" job I did in taking care of Henry. Amazing indeed that we both didn't lose our minds in the process. I guess it helps a little to know what we accomplished under tremendous odds, but I also know there was not only the valley of the shadow of death but also the shadow of withholding communication, which is almost as destructive as death itself.

I know from sad experience that the human being has untapped strengths. Henry was one of these beautiful people. He could have coped, and I needed him to help me to cope too. It's a horror to cope alone, and what destroyed me was the knowledge that he was probably doing the same thing to protect me.

And so our chapter of life is closed, but "the memories linger on." This is as it should be, and the good memories sustain one. There is always, however, an epilogue that must be written to evaluate the balance sheet of life. If the book of life is closed with truth among the protagonists, there can be real acceptance. If there is deception, the work of grief is that much harder, and the one who is left bereft must do it alone.

Since life is short, we must make the most of it. We sift out the important from the unimportant. Truth is important and supportive. Deception is destructive and makes acceptance harder to achieve.

I am ready to start a new chapter of life, but it is only because of coming to grips with the truth of why this was impossible until now that I am able to do so.

And now that I've told it like it was and like it is, I must tell it like it should be. There must be a coordinated program to help the dying and the bereaved. I couldn't honestly vent my rage, because whom was I to blame? It has taken lots of introspection and retrospection to realize what was so blatantly evident. It is a rage against the system. And that comes to the real purpose of this dissertation. It is all there before us. We have dedicated doctors, nurses, social workers, psychologists, psychiatrists, and others selflessly giving of themselves but not knowing what the other is doing and thinking. Let's pull them all together as an interdisciplinary team and open the subject of death. Serving the needs of the dying, the bereaved, and the caregivers should be the goal of this team. Otherwise everyone loses in this game where there are no winners and the stakes are high.

When Henry had had the optimum radiation and chemotherapy (I lived in his hospital room for three months), his doctor said, "I think it is time for you to go to a nursing home." I shall never forget the look of disbelief and terror in my husband's eyes as we heard those words. I immediately assured Henry and the doctor that this was out of the question, and, although I had a fractured leg that wouldn't heal because I was on it constantly, we managed a home care program that was enviable.

When he was discharged, life-saving blood was denied because we had already used 40 pints. I had learned to be a very competent nurse taking care of all his needs, and I knew that if I didn't get blood some place, then he wouldn't live to enjoy at least a little more time in the home he so desperately wanted to be in again. It was no small battle to convince the local doctor by begging and pleading for that extra blood. It was not easy to do, because I knew I was selfish in wanting to keep him alive. But I also knew that I had taken his choices away by not giving him the responsibility of decisions. And how did I know he wouldn't want it?

Then we got the miracle that made it even harder for me to let go later. He amazed every specialist as he stopped bleeding and started eating enormous amounts of food because he was no longer nauseous from chemotherapy. He gradually started to walk and talk and take an interest in life. I vividly recall the day he had a toothache and I drove him to the dear friend who is our dentist. "Abe, I want you to x-ray my whole mouth and fix all of my teeth," Henry said. I couldn't believe that he really didn't know he was dying. I learned that, although our hope system changes as we bargain for less, the looking forward must be ever present for meaningful life, whether it be years, months or days. Being in his own home gave him the opportunity to listen to his precious music, read to his grandchild, and take short rides in the car. We visited friends or our favorite hamburger or pizza joint. He ate in the car while wearing his bathrobe, but it was a change of scene and a lift to the spirit.

Henry was able to plan the menus as I cooked his favorite foods. Our den, which is on street level, was equipped with hospital bed, rocker, television, and later with commode and wheelchair. This was infinitely better than being isolated in a bedroom.

We had a few favorite people pay us short visits. A glass of wine and dessert always helped. His sense of humor sustained us all when the gloom would be coming through. The doctor and later our home nurse marveled at our coping in the face of what lay ahead. "Never compare this life of quality with someone else's quantity," was what I kept hearing from them, but it is small comfort when the loneliness sets in.

Yes, seven months at home were worth the trials and stresses. When it could be no more, the loss was even greater because I had deluded myself into believing that we had escaped the inevitable. Then the fall is even harder to accept.

Indeed the doctors admitted learning a lot from us, and I was commended for doing a Herculean job. It was Herculean because there was no support from a team. When Henry died, the local doctor, who kept telling me how worried he was about what was going to happen to me, did not come until 4½ hours later. He then insensitively said as an excuse, "My patients die in hospitals where they belong."

He was wrong. The closest place I found to home was St. Christopher's Hospice, where, two years after Henry's death, I traveled to see this stopover on one's journey through life. I knew there had to be a better way than the floundering of our traditional hospitals.

Quality home care can and should be available. There are some prerequisites that could make it much easier for the caregiver. The first and foremost is support, not only for the patient, but also for the family and spouse. How I needed help so that I wouldn't have to go in the car, find a quiet road, and scream until my throat hurt. I thought I was losing my mind at the time, but I know now that this escape valve helped me to keep my sanity.

When my father died suddenly five weeks before my husband, I had to make all kinds of complicated arrangements to leave my sick husband and go to the funeral in Florida. I felt as though I was the protagonist in a bad soap opera. When I saw my mother, everyone said those ugly words again, "Control yourself." Why, when we should have been allowed to weep in each other's arms? What is sad is that these people honestly thought that they were helping us, but it was their hangups that we were forced to satisfy.

Yes, I have grown a lot in these years. I have learned to overcome a loneliness that is not the same as being alone. It is the constant aching and yearning for someone to share with and care with. It is a marasmus that destroys the very spirit. It is a disease that has a remedy, and yet the very ones who can dispense the medication—warmth and understanding—are the ones who withhold (unwittingly or not) this life-saving antidote. It can't be bottled and it can't be bought, but like a smile, it is also beneficial to the giver. Too often, because each one is so busy, one is not sensitive to the needs of others. Yet these very needs are what the distress signals are all about. Stroke me, care for me, don't let me sink into despair. I need to know that I count and that there is a receptive shoulder to help through the grieving process.

Yes, I can thank Henry for this growing. If I had not sought some answers to the perplexing question, I might never have found the path toward helping the dying and the bereaved. Morbid? This is the response of the unknowing. I should say not. It has given me a heightened awareness of life. It has helped me discover that the needs of the bereaved are equally as important as those of the dying. This discovery can lead only to an emergence of self that was sublimated at a time when supportive help was denied.

As a teacher, I have become perceptive to the needs of children who face grief or, more aptly, don't face grief. There are lots of changes that must be promulgated in our death-denying society so that we can truly know the full meaning of life as it runs out.

♨♨♨ 13

Sexual Problems of the Terminally Ill

Lois Jaffe

Our relationship now is more that of strangers because of hospital separation. His sexual desires have diminished because our thoughts are dominated by the cancer and his impending death. The disease, however, is not repulsive to me. I've had no urge to escape from his touch as other wives have talked about. We still enjoyed sex until he was unable to perform. This was a major frustration to him and made him feel less a man and more the invalid. The frustrations in our lives caused by his illness I'm sure would be eased if we were still sexually bound and still "one." Knowing I could ease his tensions of the day at the office by loving him sexually is such a contrast with knowing I can do nothing now to ease his frustrations when he is dying. He now feels we are on opposite sides of the fence. I'm sure it's because I cannot convince him by words or actions here in the hospital. He feels his masculinity is gone and our "oneness" is gone. For 33 years, I took our loving for granted and assumed it would always be there. . . . It may sound like we were forever in bed, but sex is so much more than physical. Even talking on the phone, sitting across from each other reading, being in a crowd, even being hundreds of miles apart, we felt the union.

These are the words of a wife of a long-term hospitalized patient with brain cancer. She is a member of a group I conduct weekly on

This paper was published in *The Sexually Oppressed,* ed. H. Gochros, and is reprinted here with the permission of the publisher, Association Press (1977), and the editor.

109

an oncology unit for cancer and leukemia patients and their families. These encounters provide an opportunity for sharing feelings of anger, sadness, frustration, and fear and for learning from one another how better to cope with facing death. Her description captures the essence of the sexual problems facing the terminally ill and their loved ones.

I myself have been an acute leukemia patient for the last 28 months of my 47 years of life. In my work as death educator and family therapist, as well as in my role as patient, I have become convinced that the area of sexual problems with regard to the terminally ill constitutes a "double whammy" and thus has been enveloped in silence. There is little discussion in the literature about the fact that sexual expression is generally denied or severely compromised in situations involving terminal illness and impending interpersonal loss (Barton, 1972; Davis, 1974).

Death arouses the most basic underlying anxiety that every human being must face. The fear of the unknown is paralleled only by the fear of being cut off from life before fulfilling one's potential. Death anxiety is exacerbated by the invisibility of personal dying in our society. Eighty percent of us die in institutions, and thus we are unrehearsed in ways of interacting with those facing death, or those who are left behind. Confronting death generates more anguish and fear than any other area of human behavior. Caregivers are no different from anyone else; facing a dying person means facing one's own mortality—a realization which makes even the hardiest of souls begin to twitch. Sexuality is the only other area to engender a comparable degree of discomfort, confusion, and resistance, particularly when it must be handled by clinicians. This combination of sexuality with terminality constitutes a double-barrelled taboo.

Since sexuality and death represent the beginning and end points of life itself, anxiety is understandably heightened by their interface. For the dying patient and his loved ones, aspects of confronting death can be a classical "double-bind." In a double-bind situation, a person is faced with contradictory messages which are often concealed or transmitted on different levels. As a result of this invisibility, the individual cannot escape or effectively comment on the paradoxes which confront him (Erickson and Hyerstay, 1974). Preparing for impending death by either partner in the relationship involves accommodation to an ending, a "deadline." Sexuality, on the other hand, represents a moving forward, a perpetuation of vitality, the quintessence of the life force. Yet, despite this contrast, both experiences share a kind of "letting go." As Keleman (1974) has written: "Dying generates excitement, unformedness, unconnectedness, unknowingness. . . . Excitement is the force that connects sex and dying" (p. 27).

For the healthy spouse, the vitality of sexuality is often experienced as a direct contradiction to the finality of death. As the spouse struggles to stop thinking of the relationship as having a future, he is confronted with the dissonance between sex (a moving forward into the future) and death (an end in the present). Rather than face this clash, the healthy partner may choose not to interact sexually with the patient, and may possibly seek sexual activity with a new partner as an antidote to loss and death. Either way, there is a tendency to move away sexually and emotionally from the dying patient.

For the terminally ill patient, there is the reverse of the double-bind to confront. While the healthy partner may be avoiding sex with the patient, the patient may now desire increased sexual activity with the spouse to counter death anxiety. Sexuality, as Keleman (1974) points out, is almost a training for dying—an intensification of the dying process and a rehearsal for the dying event.

The orgastic state that produces feelings of ecstasy is a surrendering to the involuntary and to the unknown. Orgasm requires giving ourselves over to what is occurring in us. . . . The orgastic state also produces feelings of dying, raises fears of dying, because the social awareness may be threatened by the involuntary (p. 119).

The terminally ill patient holds in his possession a double-edged sword. He can either become revitalized by the intensity that comes with confronting death, thus making him more sexually aware and responsive, or he can become so frightened by the prospect of death that any stirring up of that anxiety, as in an orgasmic "letting go," may move him into an "asexual" state. It is my belief that the direction a patient chooses is largely determined by: (1) his previous experiences with sex and death; (2) the presence or absence of pain; (3) his treatment as "one of the living" rather than as a dying patient;

and (4) his perception of hope for being able to live a full and meaningful life in whatever time he has left.

Given this conceptual framework for viewing the sexual problems of the terminally ill patient and others significant to him, let us now examine the predisposing, precipitating, and perpetuating factors which make this content area so necessary and vital for intervention. By using this primary prevention approach, recommendations can then be made for therapeutic strategies.

Factors Related to the Sexual Problems of the Terminally Ill

Predisposing Factors

If one looks at the meaning of death developmentally, it is easy to understand why people are predisposed to inordinate anxiety when handling the interface between sex and death. Psychologist Maria Nagy, studying Hungarian children in the late 1940s, described three phases in the child's awareness of personal mortality as reflected in drawings and words. In stage one, the preschool child usually does not recognize the irreversibility of death, and regards it as sleep or departure. Between the ages of about five and nine, he tends to personify death as a separate figure, such as an angel or a frightening skeleton, who usually makes his rounds at night. In this second stage, death seems to be understood as final. However, an important protective feature remains: personal death can be avoided if you run faster than the Death Man, lock the door, hide from him, or trick him. Death is still external, and not general. In stage three, beginning around age nine or ten, death is recognized not only as final, but as inevitable for all (Nagy, 1959).

Given a child's concept of avoiding death by running away from the death figure, it is no wonder that many adults harbor a primitive fear that they can "catch death" from being too close to their terminally ill partner. Preconsciously, people associate death with night. Consequently, whether to sleep with a terminally ill spouse often arises as an initial conflict for the healthy partner. Case histories point to the number of spouses, who, "out of the blue," pick up and leave home after a long-term hospitalized patient finally goes into remission and/or returns home.

Reinforcing this psychological fear is the well-publicized medical research pointing to viral infection as a probable causal factor in some leukemias and other malignancies. Fear of physical transmission of the disease then compounds the spouse's anxiety. Indeed, patients with many types of malignancies, with unusually low resistance, or who are being treated with steroids are prone to secondary infections which ordinarily would not affect them. These infections can be potential hazards to people in close contact with the patient (Beeson and McDermott, 1975). Thus, the primitive fear of "catching death" is concretized by publicity regarding possible viral etiology of malignancies, as well as by the reality factor of transmissible secondary infections.

Another predisposing factor to inordinate anxiety regarding sex and death is the manner in which parents have handled these topics during the patient's childhood. When parents have been dishonest or evasive in dealing with sex and/or death, "closed communication" around the issue results. When terminal illness occurs—a time when openness is so necessary to avoid isolation and abandonment—the preestablished "conspiracy of silence" is only exacerbated (Zeligs, 1967). Also, if a woman is socialized to believe that sexuality is unimportant, "wrong," useful only for procreation, then she may experience relief at being "exempted" from this felt burden. Obviously, the quality of one's sexuality prior to terminality determines the quality as well as the quantity of sex after diagnosis.

Precipitating Factors

Even if a patient has not been predisposed by noxious developmental experiences related to sex and death, the triggering event of the terminal illness and its concomitants invariably precipitates sexual adjustments. These associated factors include numerous drugs, including severe chemotherapy, radiation, body disability. Yet, when it comes to treating the whole person, the medical team has devoted little or no attention to how a patient's sexuality may be altered or denied during the acute or chronic phases of terminal illness. Drugs, procedures, and conditions that can modify the physical or emotional aspects of sexuality are seldom, if ever, discussed with patients, their spouses, or families (Jacobson, 1974).

Medical Aspects Sexual dysfunction can result from many types of physical disorders along with the emotional reactions associated with illness (Masters and Johnson, 1970). It is important to distinguish anatomic and physiological changes from the related psychosocial effects.

Certain hematologic diseases, such as acute and chronic leukemia and Hodgkin's Disease, or their treatment, can in and of themselves cause sexual impotence. Other organic conditions associated with malignancies may decrease sexual function. These include diseases of the nervous system, surgery of the pelvic region, and endocrine disorders. None of these conditions, however, regularly destroy all sexual function.

Nervous system malignancies With regard to brain and spinal cord tumors, sexual function is more vulnerable than are the other autonomic functions of urination and defecation. In the male, orgasm and ejaculation are almost always destroyed by a complete upper motor neuron lesion, although erections are preserved. With a complete lower motor neuron lesion, erections are less frequent, but ejaculation and orgasm may occur. Bors and Comarr (1960) conclude that, with incomplete lesions, whether upper or lower, erection occurs in over 90 percent, and ejaculation and orgasm may be preserved in 32 to 70 percent of patients. They also state that interest in the other sex and desire for intercourse (or regret of impotence) are present in all male patients with spinal cord lesions. There has been much less research on the sexual behavior of women with neurologic disorders. In these cases, women's libido seems to depend on various psychodynamic factors, as well as their age, and appears to be less constant than in males (Ford and Orfirer, 1967).

Diseases That Mutilate Diseases such as cancer of the rectum and colon not only cause deterioration in bodily processes, but also result in the mutilation and deformation of the body. Consequently, the usual forms of sexual functioning may be diminished or destroyed. Radical surgery employed to prolong life may cause sexual impotence in the male, because the nerves of erection are particularly vulnerable to trauma in the dissection of the rectum and the prostate. The average incident of this dysfunction is 76 percent (Jacobson, 1974). Regardless of age, men scheduled to undergo such surgery should be apprised of the possibility of impotence afterwards. The availability of a willing and able sexual partner is the most important consideration in continuing sexual activity before and after surgery. Amputation of the penis as treatment for carcinoma is also sexually disabling; yet patients have reported satisfactory sexual lives following plastic surgical reconstruction of the penis (Barton, 1972).

The female cancer patient also presents special needs. An operation on her genitals, breasts, or reproductive organs can be an emotionally traumatic experience. Surgery in these areas often threatens a woman's self-image, making her feel a less than complete female, and symbolically signifying the end of all sexual sensation. Sexual dysfunction in these cases appears to be primarily psychologically based. Women who had radical vulvectomies performed, with total removal of the clitoris, were repeatedly orgasmic in coitus, and felt that their sexual responsiveness was existent to the same degree as before surgery (Daly, 1971).

Endocrine Disorders The main endocrine disorder associated with sexual dysfunction is diabetes milleitus. The incidence of erectile impotence in men of all ages with this disorder is two to five times higher than in the general population (Ford and Orfirer, 1967). Retrograde ejaculation is also not uncommon in diabetes. Diabetes is sometimes a secondary reaction to severe physiological stress that is often a concomitant of various malignancies and to prolonged steroid treatment sometimes used in cancer therapy. It is interesting to note that in a textbook on diabetes, the authors state: "Libido usually persists. . . . Effective therapy includes a sympathetic understanding on the part of the physician and a highly individualized approach to each patient" (Ellenberg and Rifkin, 1962, p. 337).

Effects of Drugs The effects of drugs on sexuality are generally better documented and understood for males than for females. This is partly due to the fact that the male response of erection and ejaculation is more visible and quantifiable than the lubrication and swelling in the female.

Central nervous system depressants, including alcohol, barbiturates, and sedatives, do not have a specific effect on the sex centers. However, small doses of sedatives may temporarily remove sexual inhibitions, while larger doses depress all behavior, including sex. Chronic abuse of sedatives seems to generally diminish sexual functioning. Narcotics, used to control pain, seem to reduce the sex drive specifically. However, this finding is based more upon anecdotal report than on systematically controlled study (Kaplan, 1974).

Firmer evidence supports the finding that androgens, often used in treating breast cancer, stimulate sex centers in both males and females. When phenothiazines are used to control nausea induced by chemotherapy, they can cause "dry" ejaculation to occur. This phenomenon is due to the peripheral autonomic action on the internal vesical sphincter, which causes semen to empty into the bladder instead of the urethra. Antianxiety drugs which are also muscle relaxants probably have no direct sexual effects, but sexual interest may increase as a reflection of diminished anxiety. Muscle-relaxing effects may account for the rare orgasm disturbances which are reported (Kaplan, 1974).

Effects of body changes Body changes which alter appearance and functioning will influence feelings of self-worth, and consequently exert a profound effect on sexual behavior. Extreme weight loss is generally a concomitant of malignancy. Chemotherapy frequently causes hair loss, a devastating blow to the patient's self-image, as well as a traumatizing symbol of pervasive impending losses. Such changes in the patient's appearance can be repugnant to the spouse, causing a further spiraling downward of sexual interest. Patients may use sex to deny their illness. In order to ward off feelings of loss and "asexuality," they may make sexual demands on the spouse which are quite inconsistent with former patterns in their relationship. This attempted overcompensation often meets with failure, which then triggers even more frantic efforts at denial.

Loss of sexual function due to medical factors in terminal illness is less extensive than is often assumed (Ford and Orfirer, 1967). Nonetheless, a self-fulfilling prophecy persists on the part of the patient, spouse, and caregiver; a terminally ill individual will neither be interested nor able to function effectively in sex. This assumption may have evolved from people's association of cancer with pain, such that mates try to spare their loved ones any additional discomfort. Yet this belief is not necessarily valid, for severe pain occurs in less than 15 percent of cancer patients (Exton-Smith, 1961). Thus, emotional reactions of the patient, family, and caregiver are as important in precipitating sexual dysfunction as the illness itself (Ford and Orfirer, 1967).

Anticipatory Grief An important aspect of terminal illness is designated "anticipatory grief": any grief occurring prior to rather than at the time of or following the loss (Aldrich, 1974; Schoenberg, Carr, Kutscher, Peretz, and Goldberg, 1974). One might expect a natural disengagement to occur at the same pace on the part of both the patient and spouse. As the former readies himself to "let go," the latter not only is preparing to "let go" of the patient, but may also be seeking new attachments and investments for the future. While this parallel disengagement generally occurs, the patient and his mate are frequently "out of sync" with regard to their individual experiencing of the stages of dying (Kübler-Ross, 1969). Continual confrontation in his hospital environment with the reality of impending death facilitates the patient's move toward acceptance, a part of anticipatory grief. Meanwhile, the healthy spouse may insist on denying reality, and consequently feel betrayed and resentful when the patient does not embrace his own hope for a miracle. This reaction often occurs when couples have been fused in their relationship, continually presenting a "united front" and unable to tolerate any differences between them. Being "out of sync" in the dying process can then cause an irreparable rift between them.

Clinical observations indicate that overt anticipatory grief does not consistently accelerate in degree as the loss approaches. As a matter of fact, the longer a patient is in remission, leading a normal life, the harder it is for the patient and spouse to "keep in touch" with the reality of impending death. The constant balance and flow between denial (forestalling anticipatory grief work) and acceptance (facilitating anticipatory grief work) may prevent a linear acceleration of anticipatory grief over time (Aldrich, 1974).

Long-term hospitalization, generally accompanied by sexual deprivation, may precipitate problems for either partner. The terminally ill patient generally believes that his mate is understanding and accepting of the imposed abstinence. To the contrary, however, the spouse often experiences lowered self-esteem and depression. Anger may be engendered, and expressed directly as chronic irritability, or indirectly in the form of seductive behavior toward others. Forced resignation and hopelessness may characterize some situations (Barton, 1972).

Ill health may also be a concomitant of separation for the spouse. A recent study (Chester, 1973) indicates that continuing absence of a husband as well as loss of a husband appears to precipitate ill-health in 85 percent of women who were studied in a state of psychosocial transition. Other studies (Marsden, 1969; Beikman, 1969) confirm this proneness to ill health during the periods of anticipatory grief and bereavement. These findings point to the obvious need for society to furnish such individuals with social support systems.

Severe relationship problems may occur if a patient who has been considered terminally ill does not die as predicted. Paradoxically, both partners may experience a sense of letdown with the shift in prognosis. As Peretz (1970) has pointed out: "Even the loss of an old, familiar symptom as a result of medical intervention can result in unpleasant feeling states when the symptom has provided degrees of secondary gain and control over aspects of the environment" (p. 5). In particular, the healthy spouse may be angry. Having worked through his anticipatory grief, and emotionally buried the person, he lacks the reserves to begin the relationship again. Or, he may fear getting close because of the threat of having to endure the pain of anticipated loss once again. The former patient must shift his role identity from that of a terminally ill to a healthy individual. Whatever sexual estrangement may have occurred in the course of the illness may now be compounded by these major adjustments (Fellner, 1973).

Double-bind Communication As well as the dissonance between sexuality and death, the terminally ill patient is confronted by double-bind communication patterns regarding his impending death. All too often, people close to the patient emit incongruent verbal and nonverbal messages in their attempt to conceal the patient's terminal status from him. These efforts are futile and misguided; managing a host of contradictory cues is virtually impossible, especially since most dying patients suspect and/or want to know the truth (Avorn, 1973; Feifel, 1963; Glaser and Strauss, 1965; Kelly and Frieson, 1950; Kübler-Ross, 1969). The double-bind process triggers a brutal set of social interactions which can be destructive to the patient in all areas of his life, including sexual function (Erickson and Hyerstay, 1974).

Going along with the charade will cost the patient as much psychological energy as it does others around him. The dissonance between what the patient hears and what he senses leads him to question his own perception of reality. Cut off from access to valid information concerning his condition, he fills in the gaps with his own fantasies and fears. As a result of his own helplessness and frustration in the double-bind situation, the patient may respond to others with misinterpretations and exhibit little empathy for them. His constricted and inappropriate emotional behavior serves to estrange him even further from his partner.

This "death dishonesty" is often an overlay of the sexual dishonesty which comprises many couples' *modus vivendi*. When communication patterns have been closed in general, and have been deceptive with regard to sexuality, then dishonesty about death will compound the emotional estrangement. Regardless of the quality of communication before the illness, a patient will withdraw into apathy if he realizes that trusted family members have contributed to the deception concerning his impending death (Strauss and Glaser, 1970).

Perpetuating Factors

The hospital environment is pivotal in perpetuating the sexual problems of the terminally ill. At a time when intimate human relationships are most necessary, the typical hospital design deters any nurturing of bonds between mates. Rarely is there a private room for patients to share intimacies with loved ones. The demand for conjugal visits for prisoners has been voiced more strongly than the same rights for long-term hospitalized individuals. As a human being with basic needs, the patient is certainly entitled to private, tranquil conditions for lovemaking when he is able and desirous.

Diminished sexuality can be considered as a category of loss, with the potential concomitants of depression, grief, and a process of adaptation which may include suicide. Clinical impressions indicate that as one's sexuality is perceived to decline, the incidence of suicidal ideation, suicide attempts, and suicide itself increases (Leviton, 1973). A recent study found that as suicidal ideation shifted to an actual attempt, body-image and sexual self-concept worsened. Case histories of suicidal patients indicated no sexual expression for months prior to their attempt (Henderson, 1971). These findings accord with Farber's (1968) theory of suicide as a "disease of failed hope." In his conceptualization, suicide is a function of vulnerability of the personality (low state of competence) and a deprivation (threat to acceptable life conditions).

Emotional withdrawal is a facet of anticipatory grief. Its manifestation by the patient reinforces the commonly held expectation of patient, spouse, and caregiver that the sexual life of the terminal patient ends with illness. Furthermore, the patient and spouse may consider it indulgent or inappropriate to seek pleasure during this period, and both will often refrain from making sexual overtures. The healthy spouse in particular may experience guilt over having sexual desires at this time, and the lack of gratification of these needs can lead to depression. An absence of sexual feelings then derives from the grief and depression, resulting in a decreased sense of femininity or masculinity, in turn a threat to self-esteem. A vicious circle culminates in sexual dysfunction. It is not surprising that mates who become intensely depressed during the stage of anticipatory grief and lack the comfort of a fulfilling sexual relationship are among those who commonly commit suicide. Ironically, the availability of sedatives and tranquilizers from the patient's doctor, prescribed to assuage grief, often add to the suicide potential (Danto, 1974).

A patient's sexual fantasies and feelings of sexual attachment often transfer to his primary caregiver, in many ways replacing the spouse as love object. The patient's feelings of dependency lead him to perceive the doctor as an all-powerful soother of ills. This emotional investment is reinforced by the fact that, during hospitalization, a patient's body is constantly touched and tended by doctors and nurses. Touching in this framework is exempt from the usual boundaries and taboos; even children carry out sexual exploration under the guise of "playing doctor" (Frankfort, 1972). If a woman has been taught that access to her body is permitted only if love is involved, she may reduce dissonance by developing a romantic attachment to her doctor. The same process may apply to men in relation to female doctors and nurses.

Thus, the caregiver's use of tactile comfort to minimize the patient's fear and isolation strengthens that attachment. In contrast, the common fear of a spouse to touch a terminally ill patient leads to a weakening of their bond. The efforts of the caregiver are experienced in juxtaposition with the reluctance of the spouse, and thus the parallel disengagement process is reinforced.

Recommendations for Therapeutic Intervention

I now offer recommendations for intervention, based on the aforementioned factors which can predispose, precipitate, and perpetuate sexual problems for the terminally ill and their significant others.

1. Honest and open communication regarding sex and death must begin in early childhood in order to change dysfunctional societal attitudes around both issues. In terms of death experience, small losses and griefs can prepare a child for facing larger ones. For example, instead of immediately replacing a pet that has died, parents should encourage a child's expressions of grief and his reminiscences, including a burial ritual. When a death occurs in the family, its cause should be explained to the child, and its finality differentiated from the temporary nature of sleep. The open sharing of sorrow can include funeral attendance for the child,

should he so desire. A similar candor should characterize the topic of sexuality. It is hoped that honest communication in the home could transfer to a hospital setting, obviating the need for people to maintain an often unwanted charade, ultimately so destructive to intimate relationships. If double-bind communication is considered to be causal in precipitating schizophrenia (Weakland, 1960), then it would certainly appear to trigger fear, rage, and withdrawal in the terminally ill.

2. Sexual interest and activity continue to be important in the lives of a great many long-term patients. In one study of fifty-five male and female patients, over half indicated that they would have liked to discuss sexual problems prior to discharge, preferably with a like-sexed physician (Sadoughi, Leshner and Fine, 1971). Most helping profession schools give only cursory attention to sexuality and terminality. As a result, caregivers are poorly prepared to undertake frank discussions with patients and spouses about sexual problems and practices, much less about facing death. Until these anxiety-laden subjects can be comfortably handled as part of one's ongoing education, it would seem crucial to provide separate courses on sexuality and terminality at this point in curriculum development. The courses should be offered early in the curriculum, and not as a mere afterthought for in-service training. This early exposure would facilitate students' specialization and competence in the areas. Furthermore, a combined didactic-experiential approach would enable individuals to work through their own discomfort, confusion, resistance, and biases. A combined course on sexuality and terminality could synthesize these phenomena as integral parts of the natural life-cycle, rather than as subjects ridden with pathology and taboos.

3. The hospital environment must be arranged to encourage ongoing intimacy for patient and spouse at a time when abandonment is so feared. It is an ironic juxtaposition that there is isolation in hospitalization, but virtually no privacy. In any case, the privacy of a regular hospital room could be self-defeating, since it is associated with so much pain and anxiety. A "quiet room" furnished with couch, carpet, soft lights, and music is needed to counteract the usual cold hardware of hospital rooms. Such a room could replicate the home ambience which patients miss so badly, and might be used for family and conjugal visits, as well as for group counseling sessions. To further create "home connectedness" as an antidote to disengagement, patients could bring objects from home reminiscent of shared joys, including their own bed linens. A reclining lounge chair should be available in the room of every terminally ill patient, so

that a loved one can rest comfortably near a critically ill mate who needs the reassurance of a continued loving presence. Whenever possible, live-in arrangements for spouses should be made, which are not contingent on wealth, as is generally the case. The therapeutic effects of maintaining one's personal appearance are well known. The accessibility of a hairdresser in a hospital setting would do much to refurbish one's sense of looking as well as possible. Recreation also provides a means of breaking the monotony, as well as furnishing a valuable mode for social interaction. Play, like sex, is intimately related to health and life, and should be encouraged by having a recreation facility for the terminally ill and others who are meaningful to him.

4. Individual and group counseling related to sexual issues must be an ongoing part of total patient care. Any medical workup should include an evaluation of sexual functioning, determined by a sexual history as developed by Wahl (1967). Because the spouse is so often ignored in the treatment process, yet is so vital in giving support to the patient, total care should embrace the patient, spouse, and family from the beginning. Consequently, in the early stages of the illness, sexual problems may be touched upon briefly, in the form of anticipatory guidance, by indicating how sexual drive or performance may be temporarily reduced by drugs, fatigue, etc. Once the patient is over the acute stage of the illness and able to return home, if only for short visits, the clinician should include sexuality in a list of other topics, such as return to work and living arrangements. Later, he may ease the way for the patient and/or spouse to disclose any concerns by a comment such as: "Now that you're home, I expect that you are finding your relationship somewhat different." This statement also reduces threat by implying that their problems are not unique. A most important task for the practitioner is to ascertain the meaning of sexuality in both personal and interpersonal terms for the patient and spouse. When sexuality has played a major role in a person's overall identity, more difficulties can be anticipated, especially if impairment or deprivation of sexual function are involved. Loss of a sexual outlet often precipitates a reactive depression, which is then exacerbated by avoidance of the topic. A further area of avoidance is that of counseling the elderly about sexuality. An individual over 65 years of age, terminally ill, and having sexual concerns is a victim of a "triple whammy." Age is no barrier to a continued sexual life, and when all intimacy is denied the elderly, inappropriate sexual expression may occur (Weinberg, 1971).

As I have implied throughout this article, a team approach to handling the issues of sexuality and terminality is almost mandatory. Much loneliness is engendered by hospitalization, particularly at night. Thus, caregivers, whether they be doctors, nurses, clergy, or social workers, should be interchangeably available to the patient and spouse as anxieties arise. Also, instead of becoming surrogates for the spouse, practitioners should encourage mates to touch the patient frequently.

Group counseling is particularly effective in eliciting patient-spouse concerns. It should be a regular, ongoing group, where feelings can be ventilated, information shared and clarified, and coping behavior modeled. The gamut of behavioral approaches to sexual counseling that have been researched and documented could be used. These include the therapeutic use of masturbation ("self-exploration"), fantasies, and the regenerating use of the vibrator for women (Annon, 1973). Counseling can also focus on techniques to remedy sexual dysfunction (Masters and Johnson, 1970; Kaplan, 1974), and coital positions that are more comfortable for the disabled (Goldberg, 1960; Romano, 1973a and b). Groups are settings conducive for discussing sex, since most people have had some experience in peer-group disclosure on the topic (Romano, 1973). Thus, groups can be enabling and educational, providing an opportunity for the modeling of desirable behaviors within a nonthreatening context. The support of other individuals facing similar problems engenders hope for being able to live a full, meaningful life in whatever time is left.

Terminal illness and impending loss can lead to an intensification of life and serve as a stimulus for a new and richer phase of development. Certainly the common assumption that the sexual life of the terminally ill ends with their diagnosis is not borne out by research or clinical observation. Although this attitude is rarely verbalized, its existence is reflected in caregivers' avoidance of the subject. The available literature indicates that sexuality continues as an important part of many patients' lives, although drive and rate of performance may be reduced. Today, such patients survive longer and with better functional capacity than ever before. Once past the acute stage of illness, they begin to search for a new equilibrium not centered on sickness or disability. It seems both appropriate and necessary to facilitate life-promoting sexual relationships as a factor in any treatment program. As Toynbee has so poignantly written:

Love cannot save life from death, but it can fulfill life's purpose.

References

Aldrich, G. 1974. "Some Dynamics of Anticipatory Grief." In *Anticipatory Grief*, eds. B. Schoenberg, A. C. Carr, A. Kutscher, D. Peretz, and I. Goldberg, pp. 3–9. New York: Columbia University Press.

Annon, J. 1973. "The Therapeutic Use of Masturbation in the Treatment of Sexual Disorders." In *Advances in Behavior Therapy,* eds. R. Rubin, J. Brody, and J. Henderson. New York: Academic Press.

Avorn, J. 1973. "Beyond Dying." *Harper's,* March, 56–64.

Barton, D. 1972. "Sexually Deprived Individuals." *Medical Aspects of Human Sexuality,* February, 88–97.

Beeson, P. and W. McDermott. 1975. *Textbook of Medicine.* Philadelphia: W. B. Saunders.

Beikman, P. 1969. "Spouseless Motherhood, Psychological Stress and Physical Morbidity." *Journal of Health and Social Behavior* 10.

Bors, E. and A. Comarr. 1960. "Neurological Disturbances of Sexual Function with Special Reference to 529 Patients with Spinal Cord Injury." *Urological Survey* 10:191–222.

Chester, R. 1973. "Health and Marital Breakdown: Some Implications for Doctors." *Journal of Psychosomatic Research* 17:317–21.

Daly, M. 1971. "The Clitoris as Related to Human Sexuality." *Medical Aspects of Human Sexuality* 5:80.

Danto, B. 1974. "Drug Ingestion and Suicide During Anticipatory Grief." In *Anticipatory Grief,* ed. B. Schoenberg et al., pp. 311–14.

Davis, K. 1974. "Eros and Thanatos: The Not-So-Benign Neglect." *Texas Report on Biology and Medicine* 32:43–48.

Ellenberg, M. and H. Rifkin. 1962. *Clinical Diabetes Mellitus.* New York: McGraw-Hill.

Erickson, R. and B. Hyerstay. 1974. "The Dying Patient and the Double-bind Hypothesis." *Omega* 5:287–98.

Exton-Smith, A. 1961. "Terminal Illness in the Aged." *Lancet* 2:305.

Farber, M. 1968. *Theory of Suicide.* New York: Funk and Wagnalls.

Feifel, H. 1963. "Death." In *Taboo Topics,* ed. N. Farberow. New York: Atherton.

Fellner, C. 1973. "Family Disruption after Cancer Cure." *American Family Physician* 8:169–72.

Ford, A. and A. Orfirer. 1967. "Sexual Behavior and the Chronically Ill Patient." *Medical Aspects of Human Sexuality* 1:51–61.

Frankfort, E. 1972. *Vaginal Politics.* New York: Bantam.

Glaser, B. and A. Strauss. 1965. *Awareness of Dying.* Chicago: Aldine.

Goldberg, M. 1960. "What Do You Tell Patients Who Ask About Coital Positions?" *Medical Aspects of Human Sexuality* December:43–48.

Henderson, J. 1971. "Competence, Threat, Hope and Self-Destructive Behavior: Suicide." Unpublished dissertation. College Park: University of Maryland.

Jacobson, L. 1974. "Illness and Human Sexuality." *Nursing Outlook* 22:1, 50–53.

Kaplan, H. 1974. *The New Sex Therapy.* New York: Brunner/Mazel.

Keleman, S. 1974. *Living Your Dying.* New York: Random House.

Kelly, W. and J. Friesen. 1950. "Do Cancer Patients Want to Be Told?" *Surgery* 27:822–26.

Kübler-Ross, E. 1969. *On Death and Dying.* New York: Macmillan.

Leviton, D. 1973. "The Significance of Sexuality as a Deterrent to Suicide Among the Aged." *Omega* 4 (2):163–74.

Marsden, D. 1969. *Mothers Alone.* London: Allen Lane.

Masters, W. and V. Johnson. 1970. *Human Sexual Inadequacy.* Boston: Little, Brown and Company.

Nagy, M. 1959. "The Child's View of Death." In *The Meaning of Death,* ed. H. Feifel. New York: McGraw-Hill.

Parkes, C. M. 1964. "Effects of Bereavement on Physical and Mental Health—A Study of the Medical Records of Widows." *British Medical Journal* 2:274.

Parkes, C. M. 1971. "Psychosocial Transitions: A Field for Study." *Social Science and Medicine* 5.

Peretz, D. 1970. "Development, Object-relationships and Loss. In *Loss and Grief,* eds. B. Schoenberg et al. New York: Columbia University Press.

Romano, M. 1973a. "Sexual Counseling in Groups." *The Journal of Sex Research* 9(1):69–78.

Romano, M. 1973b. "Sexuality and the Disabled Female." *Accent on Living,* pp. 27–35.

Sadoughi, W., M. Leshner, and H. Fine. 1971. "Sexual Adjustment in a Chronically Ill and Physically Disabled Population: A Pilot Study." *Archives of Physical Medicine and Rehabilitation* 52:311–17.

Schoenberg, B., A. C. Carr, A. H. Kutscher, D. Peretz, and I. Goldberg, eds. 1974. *Anticipatory Grief.* New York: Columbia University Press.

Schoenberg, B., A. C. Carr, D. Peretz, and A. H. Kutscher. 1970. *Loss and Grief.* New York: Columbia University Press.

Strauss, A. L. and B. Glaser. 1970. *Anguish: A Case History of a Dying Trajectory.* Mill Valley, California: Sociology Press.

Wahl, C. 1967. "Psychiatric Techniques in the Taking of a Sexual History." In *Sexual Problems: Diagnosis and Treatment in Medical Practice,* ed. C. Wahl. New York: The Free Press.

Weakland, J. 1960. "The Double-bind Hypothesis of Schizophrenia and Three-Party Interaction." In *The Etiology of Schizophrenia,* ed. D. Jackson. New York: Basic Books.

Weinberg, J. 1971. "Sexuality in Later Life." *Medical Aspects of Human Sexuality* April:216–22.

Zeligs, R. 1967. "Children's Attitudes Toward Death." *Mental Hygiene* 51:393–96.

⚘⚘⚘ 14

Case Reports

Josephine A. Lockwood

Case Report 1

The patient presented is a 22-year-old woman initially admitted to the Metropolitan Home Care Program in 1966. The patient has severe mental retardation, paralysis of left side of body, difficulty in speaking, weakness of right side of her body, and sickle cell anemia. The patient had had normal infant development and growth until the age of five years. At that time she developed weakness of the right side owing to a stroke, which was the result of her sickle cell anemia. Three years later she had a more severe stroke which resulted in the subsequent failure of mental development, as well as in the paralysis of the left side of her body. Between that time and 1972, she has had numerous episodes of sickle cell crisis requiring hospitalization.

Before her admission to Metropolitan Hospital Center's home care service she had been a patient at Willowbrook State Hospital and had developed decubitus ulcers on her back, and her condition had deteriorated. Her mother took her from Willowbrook, although psychologically and physically unable to provide the care the patient required. Since this patient's admission to Metropolitan's home care program she has been able to be maintained at home with care provided by her mother. This has required extensive counseling of the patient's mother by our social service worker, as well as by our staff psychiatrist. Housekeeping assistance was needed, since the patient's mother had three other children who also required her care. This assistance made it possible for the patient to be maintained in the commu-

128

nity. A physical therapy program was initiated and operative procedures for relief of deformities of joints were performed so that the patient was able to move with assistance from a bed to a wheelchair. At present she continues to be confined largely to a wheelchair; her mother takes her outdoors to social activities, and the home situation continues stable. Speech therapy was instituted, and the patient was able to communicate single words with the aid of a word board. With immediate treatment of any infections, sickle cell crises have been prevented to a large degree. This patient's last hospitalization was in September 1974, and previous hospitalization was two years before that. Previously she had required monthly hospitalizations.

Other supportive services that have been and continue to be provided are camp programs so that the patient has been able to participate in camp activities outside the home for two- to four-week intervals; institutionalization at Bird S. Coler Hospital for two-week intervals when and if the care of the patient becomes overwhelming to the mother; careful followup by a physician visiting the patient in the home to ensure appropriate treatment of the current infections and supervision by the hematology service at infrequent intervals to ensure stability from a hematologic point of view. At present, the patient remains stable and able to be maintained in the home. The mother continues to require supportive care and ventilation sessions, and the medical supervision delineated continues to be necessary. Physical therapy and speech therapy are no longer provided on a regular basis, since the patient is stable, but reevaluations are conducted at six- to eight-month intervals, and additional treatment has been provided when indicated.

While the prognosis in this situation remains dire, the fact that the patient has been able to be maintained with the care provided is, indeed, a success story for the ability of in-home medical, social, and nursing supervision to provide maintenance care.

Without such supervision there is no question that the home situation would have disintegrated; that the mother, who has numerous emotional problems, would not have been able to provide the necessary care; and that rehospitalization in an acute hospital setting would have occurred at very frequent intervals, with probable transfer to another chronic care setting.

Case Report 2

On August 21, 1975, a patient was discussed after referral to the Metropolitan Hospital home care service who had been a patient in the hospital from

July 5 to July 21, 1975. He had been discharged to home at that time, after which he was felt to be in need of more careful supervision in his home setting. He found great difficulty in attending outpatient department and was unable to get to a private physician for supervision of his care. His medical problems were such that he required continuing in-home medical visits. His medical diagnoses are diabetes mellitus (patient was on insulin medication and unable to administer this medication appropriately to himself), high blood pressure, and other problems that caused degeneration of mental function. He is also blind and has marked hearing difficulties. He was hospitalized on July 5 because his diabetes mellitus had gone out of control. He was sent home on insulin therapy but had difficulty in administering this medication, and his wife had difficulty in supervising his care. For this reason he was evaluated and subsequently accepted for care through delivery of home health agency services.

This patient requires extensive coordinated care with attention to a multiplicity of medical and serious home problems. Patient's wife is 65 years old and was found by the doctor from our home care program to have many medical problems. She had had a recent hospitalization because of extensive arteriosclerosis of blood vessels supplying brain areas and has periodic episodes of dizziness. In addition, she also has diabetes mellitus and a number of complications as a result of the diabetes. She has advanced arthritis of the knees and finds ambulation very difficult both because of the arthritis and because of the dizziness. Both patients require (1) nursing care supervision to ensure appropriate use of medications and renforcement of necessity for calorie-restricted diets; (2) physical therapy, especially for the wife, to ensure the maximum ability to function and minimal effort on her part in assisting her husband in his care; (3) further family evaluation, which is being conducted.

On further contact with these two patients we found that the 85-year-old parent of one has had no appropriate medical supervision over the past several years. She has been unable to get to any source of medical care and is therefore being considered for supervision in a home setting. In addition, housekeeping assistance is needed if we are to maintain these three very ill and marginally stable family members in the community. This is being evaluated further, but at present the family is receiving assistance twice weekly to help with shopping, cleaning, and laundry. A physician visits both patients at two- to three-week intervals to maintain medical stability. Laboratory evaluation for control of the diabetes mellitus is done at monthly intervals. Of note is the fact that both patients had had uncontrolled blood sugar readings during the past two months, but since acceptance on home care, both have been under adequate control. This is largely due to supervision of medication administration and instruction, and also to the appropriate provision of supportive services, such as housekeeping assistance and the availability of a person to obtain medications for all family members. Early signs of decompensation are determined by the physician or nurse on visits to this family, and all family members call if any interim problems arise.

Without a program delivering care in the home, only the husband, in this situation, would receive medical supervision. Without appropriate care of all family members the entire home situation would rapidly decompensate, and three family members would require institutional care. Needless to say, the cost of provision of home health agency services for the care and supervision of these three family members is minimal when compared with the cost of institutional care.

Case Report 3

This patient was a 56-year-old gentleman who had been admitted to Metropolitan Hospital Center for the first time in February 1974. At that time a brain tumor was discovered, and surgery was performed. It was felt that the tumor had been completely removed, and he was discharged with medications to prevent convulsions and with minimal pain medication. He was readmitted to the hospital in May 1975 because of the onset of weakness over the left side of his body. He had additional symptoms of headache and nausea and vomiting. It was felt that these represented the recurrence of the tumor, and subsequent studies indicated the same. At that time he was given a full course of radiotherapy in the hope that this could allay subsequent growth of the very malignant tumor that this patient was known to have.

Approximately one month later he again noted increasing weakness of the left side of his body, as well as recurrence of severe headaches. He was readmitted, and another course of x-ray therapy was administered. At that time he was referred for home health services. The patient was anxious to remain in the community and wanted to return home. He had been living with a friend for approximately 20 years, and this friend was concerned and more than willing to provide needed assistance and supervision. After interviews with the friend and the patient it was felt that this patient had a right to return home and that all that could be done supportively should be done to maintain him in the community for as long as possible. He was, therefore, accepted on home care, and the following services were provided: (1) Physician visits were made to the home to supervise and revise medication orders when needed, since the patient was in need of increasing amounts of narcotic medications to alleviate the severe headaches that continued. In addition to that he developed many ancillary medical problems as a result of the brain tumor, the deconditioning that occurred after his stability, complications of large dosage of narcotic medication (e.g., retention of urine and need for catheterization and supervision). (2) Occupational therapy home supervision was provided, along with assistive devices that could assist this patient in remaining ambulatory for as long as possible. The patient subsequently became limited to a wheelchair for propulsion, but for approximately three months at home he continued to be able to ambulate with the aid of a walker. He was also provided with special equipment to assist in eating, since he subsequently developed weakness of all extremities. (3) Social service supervision, counseling and visits in the home were provided to ensure that the patient's friend was able to continue the total care that subsequently became necessary. At no time did any housekeeping or any other social service supportive services become required, since the friend was able to provide all the needed care. Counseling was of great help in maintaining this patient in the home and in providing support for the patient's friend. (4) Psychiatric consultation and interpretation to the patient's friend were done by our staff psychiatrist. In addition to this our psychiatrist worked closely with all staff so that proper provision of care and interpretation would be able to be provided. (5) Care during in-hospital stays and carryover into the home were coordinated through the physician on the home care staff. (6) Visiting nurse service supervision and instruction in administration of medications were delivered. The patient required increasing amount of intramuscular narcotics as his disease progressed. His friend was able and willing to administer these medications, and the supervision and instruction in the administration of this medicine were provided through this service.

In summary we are presented with a patient who at a young age developed a malignant brain tumor. Despite all treatment the tumor progressed, and the patient became increasingly reliant on supportive services. The provision and supervision of such services were carried out through medical and affiliated medical services, as well as by a friend who might be regarded as closer than a family member. Without such care, this patient would not have been able to return home after his second hospitalization. With this supervision he remained at home over the next three months, after which he was admitted to the hospital on the morning of one particularly difficult day. He expired several hours later. The patient's desire was to have remained at home until death, and his wish had, for all intents and purposes, been fulfilled. The costs for care by the aforementioned medical care personnel were certainly less than those that would have accrued if this patient had been transferred to an institution such as a terminal care facility or a chronic care hospital. In addition, recurrent hospitalizations were not required, since problems could be taken care of when they arose at home.

Part III

Home Care Services

⚘⚘⚘ 15

Twenty-Five Years
of Home Care Services
Celia Moss Hailperin

Home Care Beginnings

As researched by Sidney M. Bergman, former executive director of Montefiore Hospital of Western Pennsylvania, the earliest accessible record of a home care program was in Gheel, Belgium, in the fourteenth century for patients with emotional symptoms. This still operative program selects families in the community who care for these patients as participating members of the family.

In the United States the earliest development of home care appears to have been established in 1796 at the Boston Dispensary for medical care to the "sick poor." It was based on the following:

1. The sick, without being pained by a separation from their families, may be attended and relieved in their own homes.
2. The sick can in this way be assisted at a less expense to the public than in any hospital.
3. Those who have seen better days may be comforted without being humiliated, and all the poor receive the benefits of a charity, the more refined as it is the more secret.

137

This program still operates on a more extended scale.

In 1875, Boston University School of Medicine and the Massachusetts Homeopathic Hospital instituted a home care program that continues as part of the senior medical student's education experience. In 1936 a similar program was developed at the University of Vermont, with other schools of medicine, such as the University of Pennsylvania, establishing like educational programs.

However, the development of "hospital-based coordinated home care programs" had its beginning in 1945 with the vision of Dr. E. M. Bluestone, executive director of New York's Montefiore Hospital, by translation of services of the modern hospital to the home of the patient. This was, indeed, a contemporary model of a traditionally sound basic idea, which developed a team concept, demonstrated the validity of the social worker's inclusion on this team, and emphasized the importance of her or his interrelated home care contribution along with those of the physician and nurse.

On the basis of this program, the Montefiore Hospital of Western Pennsylvania began its home care program with a small, limited number of cases, to determine whether such a modality would be realistic in Pittsburgh. The executive director, Sidney Bergman, was enthusiastic and supportive, despite the fact that budgetary provisions were withheld.

A situation of particular relevance occurred during the early days of the program. As the director of the social service department, I had noticed a young man pacing back and forth from the open door of my office. He would read the sign above my door and then hurriedly move on to the elevator across the hall. After several such occasions, I approached him and asked if I could help. He thought that no one could, but he came in and sat down. With his head in his hands, he talked about being deluged with troubles. His 30-year-old wife, the mother of their two children aged one and five, had recently had surgery for the second time in six months. Her diagnosis of metastatic intestinal carcinoma had had optimal treatment according to the surgeon, who had advised the patient that she could go home for the three to four months until her death. How could she go home? Who would care for her? What about the children? The husband spoke of the debts that had accrued over the past six months. There were no family or close friends in the area. He worked as an accountant in the local VA regional office. Through his veteran's benefits, after his discharge from military service, he had made a down payment on his home. Payments were in arrears. Unexpected medical and housekeeping expenses had mounted far beyond his financial resources. A single sister, living in California, had offered to come to help, if her transportation could be arranged. He was unable to meet such expense. He wanted to keep the family together, but how?

The thought occurred to me that this situation was truly a potential for home care. I asked him to return in two days. In the meantime I would look into possible resources to help alleviate the difficulties. Taking the matter to my administrator, I suggested this as a potential home care case if the wife's physician would agree to make home visits and the hospital would provide necessary equipment and supplies. We talked about other needs—nursing primarily, and a telephone call to the Visiting Nurse Association brought a quick response. The local Cancer Society agreed to provide dressings and medications, and our women's auxiliary agreed to pay the sister's transportation from California, if she were still willing to come. The social service director would coordinate these activities. When the plan was presented to the patient and her husband, they were very relieved. The husband called his sister from my office and discussed the entire situation with her. She realized this was not an ordinary visit, and that she would arrange to stay at least six months, if necessary, to care for the children, cook, and do what was necessary with the supports set up by the hospital. Within two days, patient was discharged following her relative's arrival and the delivery of a hospital bed, bedside unit, drugs, dressings prescribed by the physician, and a plan for the physician's and nurse's visits.

She lived 10 months. During this time she was readmitted to the hospital briefly twice for blood transfusions and a third time, shortly before her death. She was able to participate in many usual activities with her loving family. With the continued home care supports, they were all better able to cope with their anxieties, experiencing a quality of living for the dying patient and those around her.

We kept a record of this and several other home care situations, which Mr. Bergman, the hospital administrator, used to illustrate the potentials of home care. He spoke before many community groups about this, never realizing that one such address would bring the opportunity for a demonstration in hospital home care.

In 1951, with an invitation from the Sarah Mellon Foundation, he submitted a three-year proposal that emphasized, in addition to services, a research design, including a control group, to monitor the efficacy of this program.

Following this private foundation grant, which was extended to four years, the Heart Institute of the National Institutes of Health and the Pennsylvania State Health Department awarded a three-year grant to study a group of congestive heart patients in relation to home care service. This, again, was designed with a research and a service emphasis and resulted in a published report entitled "Evaluation of Congestive Heart Patients for Home Care Services."

Of interest is the timing of a study in 1960, by Dr. Cecil Sheps, of the health needs of the Jewish aging in Pittsburgh. His findings indicated the desirability of the local United Jewish Federation's support to the hospital for appropriate aged patients. The Federation has continued since that time to contribute toward this program. In 1961, with the services satisfactorily demonstrated, the board of directors of Montefiore Hospital of Western Pennsylvania created and approved a budget for a department of home care.

With the identification of this home care program as one of five national training centers for home care and related activities, a series of educational programs was developed through seven years of grant support by the Public Health Service. A steady stream of individual physicians, nurses, and social workers, as well as groups of separate and interdisciplinary professionals, came from several states to share this experience. Pittsburgh's Montefiore home care staff engaged in a variety of educational programs, both at their home base through institutes and conferences, and with travel to many other areas to help in initiating coordinated home care.

The Five-Year Project: Hospital Services for the Child at Home

In 1962 all the resources of the well-established home care program of Montefiore Hospital of Western Pennsylvania were made available to include a population of chronically ill children, identified within the geographic limits of the program. The published report of this five-year service and research demonstration was presented to the then-sponsoring agencies—Children's Bureau, Social Rehabilitation Service, Department of Health, Education, and Welfare; Commonwealth of Pennsylvania's Department of Health; and the Montefiore Hospital of Western Pennsylvania.

Continuing evaluation of this pediatric endeavor was related to identifying the needs of and services required for chronically ill children under comprehensive medical management and the comparative similarity to and differences from the needs of and services for adults served by the home care program. At the end of the five-year period, significant facts emerged supporting the concept of continuity of care, as well as the advantages of a family-centered approach by an interdisciplinary team of pediatrician, nurse, and social worker.

Cases included a wide range of medical diagnoses, as well as socioeconomic backgrounds. Ages of patients ranged from 2 weeks through 17 years. All medical problems in this study were considered to be chronic if anticipated to be of more than three months' duration. That the mother or mother-substitute be emotionally and physically able and willing to care for the child at home was another criterion. Children, to be home care patients, were not required to be bedridden, so long as their condition required continuing medical management and they could not be brought *comfortably* to the pediatrician's office or outpatient department.

At the end of the five-year period, approximately 2,000 children had been surveyed, with less than 25 percent being potential home care candidates. As in most new medical care programs, the first year brought many inappropriate requests unrelated to home care because of existing gaps in services. This program also included several terminally ill children with varying diagnoses. For many of the families of these children, their months, weeks, or days of living were enhanced through these supports.

These developments had been initiated before the 1965 federal legislation mandated by the 89th Congress in their passage of Titles XVIII and XIX of the Social Security Amendments—Medicare and Medicaid. The exploding expectations, however, have been limited beyond the capacity of many aged and chronically ill to benefit sufficiently, because of the interpretations of this legislation.

My professional perceptions of these home care patients seemed to be reflected in a constitutional panorama. By "constitutional" I refer to Tucker and Lessa's (1940) definition:

Constitution = the sum total of the morphological, physiological, and psychological characteristics of an individual with additional variables of race, sex and age, all in large part determined by heredity but influenced in varying degrees by environmental factors, which, when integrated and expressed as a single, biological entity, fluctuate in varying degrees over a wide range of normality and occasionally cross an arbitrary boundary into "abnormality" and "pathology."

The home care patient has crossed this arbitrary boundary but has brought with him, with some modifications, all of his constitutional residuals, which he exposes to the home care team of physician, nurse, and social worker.

My perceptions of the home care patient focus on a series of dynamically, emotionally charged, colorful collages in which the chronically ill person is surrounded by and interacts with his family in his usual *familiar* environment—familiar even though his own bed may have been replaced by a hospital bed as a part of his home care services. On the premise that the family is the basic unit of health and disease, the patient in his home is psychologically as well as geographically within his primary unit of living.

To begin to paint these collages, it is necessary to sketch in some outlines of who these patients were. What were their diagnoses and prognoses, their medical and related health care needs, their ages, and their family in and out of the homes? Then we should fill in, with more subdued coloring, the background of what home care services provided appropriately in meeting identified needs.

To answer these questions, let us take a hospital's daily home care census of approximately 100 patients, of whom forty were children under the age of 17, twenty were adults between 17 and 65, and forty were adults over the age of 65. It is obvious that we were dealing primarily with youth and the aging.

As to their health problems, most had multiple diagnoses. In the adult group, more than half had some form of heart disease. Cancer and rheumatoid arthritis represented 20 percent. Patients convalescing with hip and spinal fractures made up about 5 percent, and the remaining 25 percent were patients with such long-term illnesses as emphysema, diabetes, asthma, Parkinson's disease, diverticulosis, multiple sclerosis, and cardiovascular accidents. Among the children, major diagnoses included carcinoma, scoliosis (postcorrective surgery—body casted), convulsive seizures, muscular dystrophy, arthritis, rheumatic fever, tuberculosis adenitis, asthma, Potts disease, hemophilia, hepatitis, postencephalitis, and other neurological and neuromuscular disorders.

Before discussing the staff and service requirements implied in the illnesses of these patients, it seems important to describe what was involved in this coordinated home care program. Treatment goals included use of the hospital and community resources in a wide spectrum of available services and facilities for restoration of health to maximum capacity, maintenance or improvement of physical and social functioning, and prevention of disability insofar as was possible. For those terminally ill, there was improvement of the quality of living with their families, even though death was imminent. The patient never felt abandoned.

The home care program of the Montefiore Hospital Association of Western Pennsylvania is a phase in the concept of continuity of care. It extends hospital services and facilities, augmented by community resources, to homebound patients, regardless of financial status, who are too ill to continue treatment on a regular ambulatory basis. It consists of essential elements that guarantee health standards found in the hospital. Some of these are the following:

1. Centralization of responsibility for administration. The hospital thus remains accountable for the patient's care, and the patient is assured of continuing medical management.

2. A formally structured coordinating unit composed of physicians, nurses, social workers, and clerical personnel. Additional specialties are available as indicated. Two nurses had full-time administrative assignments to the home care department—one serving as nurse liaison with adult patients also engaged in training program activities; the other was coordinating nurse liaison with the children's cases and had some research responsibility. They coordinated nursing services supplied to home care patients by the Visiting Nurse Association.
3. The multidisciplinary team, which
   a. did admission evaluation of applicants referred to the program,
   b. planned for reviews and modified individual patient need,
   c. implemented and coordinated direct patient services provided by the various professions,
   d. carried out discharge determinations, when the patient was sufficiently improved to go comfortably to his physician's office or to the outpatient department. (The patient could be readmitted to the program at any time, on the recommendation of the physician, if his condition grew worse while he was receiving home care services. To the extent that he required institutionalization, these plans were made before patients were discharged from the program.

There was also a guarantee that, when a home care patient required rehospitalization, a bed was immediately available to him, upon the request of his physician.

Dr. Victor Christopherson (1962) has suggested an orderly attempt at gauging the need of the chronically ill, which he identifies as stages of disability. This consideration also proposes potential help in pinpointing the perceptions of the patient in his key relationship in each stage. I quote these four stages of disability as a helpful backdrop in a review of the home care patients:

1. The *acute stage,* representing the initial onset when a member of the family becomes ill and an ominous diagnosis is forthcoming. Some families, in their panic, frantically seek other diagnostic sources in an attempt to reverse the inevitable prognosis. From here the patient moves on to one of the next three stages.
2. The *reconstructive stage,* referring to the period when the patient has passed the acute stage and is being treated through surgery, physical therapy, radiology, and so forth, to regain as much physical functioning as possible. Emotionally this is a critical time for the patient, for he is faced

with the implications for his future. Realistic and unrealistic perceptions on the part of both patient and family occur, as they visualize imagined and real changes in occupational, social, and sexual status. Changes in physical appearance and function may be observable. Assessment of these perceptions is significant at this time in helping establish goals of possible restoration. This is the stage when interdisciplinary activity, such as is possible in home care, can be meaningful toward rehabilitative objectives. Whereas some patients with sufficient progress are able to resume former activities, many have now reached the point of optimum benefit without return of former functioning and move on to the next stage.

3. The *plateau stage* Dr. Christopherson describes as the third phase of disability. It is assumed that all possible restorative recommendations have been tried and that the patient has reached a point of "diminutive return." Efforts are now made to sustain the optimum gains and to preserve the status quo. This is usually the most difficult period for both the patient and family. Hope for improvement diminishes with implications of physical and social confinement for the patient and overwhelming responsibility for care by the family. This is the period of heavy emotional strains in family relationships. The plateau stage, which should be interpreted as dynamically as possible, is usually of long duration and is the period for which a coordinated home care program may be very beneficial. This is the time when the family places a television set in the patient's room and finds communication with him more and more difficult as he moves into irreversible illness and the role of the dying patient.

4. The fourth phase, the *deteriorative stage,* refers to the terminal aspects of the illness where, for most, there becomes little in the way of any quality of living.

The hospital patient at home is rarely in the acute stage described here. The 100 patients referred to earlier do, however, come under the other three categories—(1) the reconstructive stage for those patients who can be sufficiently rehabilitated to return to their former way of living—sometimes healthier than their pre-home-care experience; (2) the plateau stage, representing our largest group of patients—those whose chronic illness was irreversible but whose gains could be sustained and further disability postponed and, sometimes, prevented; (3) the deteriorative stage—that of terminal illness—especially applicable to home care patients, for this modality of care can help sustain both patient and family, helping them live as they cope with difficulties inherent in terminal illness.

At both ends of the swinging pendulum, in the rehabilitative stage, patients remain on hospital home care for comparatively short periods of time. The patients in the plateau stage, where further restoration is not possible, remain on hospital home care much longer. This care prevents the frequent rehospitalizations experienced before home care. The terminal patient is at the other end of the swinging pendulum.

Dimensions of each individual's disability require study as part of their diagnostic workup. The identification of individual needs and of the most appropriate specific treatment plan for care goes beyond the diagnosis of a chronic disease.

In chronic illness, even though the disease entity may be similar, much depends on the individuals, who differ one from the other in treatment problems. In the illness itself, specific factors are relevant, such as severity of the illness, pain, progressive or stabilizing aspects, bed-confining or ambulatory requirement, extent of disability, condition at onset, length of present illness, and specific reaction to illness. Understanding a given patient so that optimum help can be offered requires a critical assessment of him as he functions in relation to his physical limitations, his interaction with those who make up his household, his employment, his leisure-time activities, and other interests.

Despite the reality of the severity of the illness, each person in his family unit uniquely organizes attitudes and perceptions toward common life crises from residues of past experience. A patient may seem hesitant to accept the dependent role concomitant with being cared for or may be suspicious of the offer of the service. Our culture, which defines adequacy as physical fitness and is work-production oriented, affects the ill person's self-image. It is needless to state that these observations imply an interdisciplinary meshing of professional understanding, as well as contributions most frequently referred to as "teamwork."

Medical progress pointed toward the preservation of life and restoration of life and function has obviously been remarkable. Having defined and determined life as a birthright, we have directed immense energy and resource to the preservation of life for all persons. We have, in effect, reversed or replaced nature's law of survival of the fittest by a moral and ethical law of survival of all, from weakest to strongest and youngest to oldest.

Inherent with this concept of life is the responsibility of preventing, when possible, or restoring, physical and social functioning to those with chronic illness or physical impairment, to the optimal function of which they are capable. Prevention and restoration, however, are only part of the overall responsibility of health and medical care. To neglect the interpersonal competency of the individual within his family is in effect to thrust him prematurely into the deteriorative and final stage of his life. Attrition can result as surely from emotional wear and tear as from physical accident or failure (LaBarre, 1954).

References

Christopherson, Y. A. 1962. "Illness and Social Functioning." Presented at Home Care Training Center, Montefiore Hospital of Western Pennsylvania. Unpublished.

LaBarre, W. 1954. *The Human Animal.* Chicago: The University of Chicago Press.

Tucker, W. B. and W. A. Lessa. 1940. "Man, A Constitutional Investigation." *Quarterly Review of Biology,* September.

𝕽𝕽𝕽 16

An Organized Home Care Program

Hanna Eichwald

"**H**ome Care" as it is known today is not a new concept. Boston City Hospital established it as early as 1780, complete with social workers and other paramedical personnel.

The program was reestablished by the City of New York in 1948. At that time certain guidelines in regard to selection and treatment of patients were set up, many of which have been modified over the years according to needs and the availability of personnel. Essentially, the program provides hospital-type treatment in the home of selected patients who are in need of the coordinated care of several disciplines. It acknowledges this need and provides for the patient to be treated in the right place, at the right time in the patient's life relative to the disease process, and by suitably effective means.

Aside from the fact that early discharge to home frees hospital beds needed for acutely ill patients, our program makes it possible for the patient to derive the full benefit of his own home, of familiar surroundings, routines, and food, and to be with concerned family members and friends. Thus, recovery is often quicker and more nearly complete, and motivation toward return to function is often better than in the impersonal hospital environment, with its perennial shortage of staff. The patient and his family (nuclear and/or ex-

148

tended) receive the psychological and emotional support they need in adjusting to chronic illness. To accomplish this, medical, paramedical, and auxiliary services are provided for the patient, and one-to-one relationships with physician, nurse, social worker, and others are established. The entire service is coordinated by a small staff of professional public health nurses, operating from within the hospital; the patient and his family thus have access to a coordinating link between them and the multiple types of professional care that might be required. In addition, a feeling of security is introduced for people who are afraid of the vastness of a large city hospital, and whose problems easily become lost in bureaucratic machinery.

Home care may be thought of as a ''hospital without walls,'' the ''extension of the hospital into the community.'' Metropolitan Hospital, whose program is described in this paper (Annual Reports, 1968–69, 1970, 1971), is a 1,000-bed municipal hospital located in East Harlem in New York City. It serves much of the indigent population of Black and Spanish Harlem, although about 20 percent of its served population are of other ethnic backgrounds. The home care daily census is 230 to 240 patients, most of whom have more than one chronic illness and multiple problems. About two-thirds of the patient population is over 65 years of age; women outnumber men about three to one. Many patients are living with their families in crowded quarters, owing to economic stress and a shortage of adequate housing, and thus the problems of old age and disease are compounded. There is often lack of privacy for patient and family, the latter sometimes including very young, as well as teenage children. Sharing sleeping facilities is common and may give rise to resentment. About 15 percent of these patients live alone, despite serious medical and functional difficulties, but they do not accept alternate plans. One basic tenet learned through the years is that a patient has the right to determine his fate, what is done to and for him and where; this right must be respected. Often it is difficult to convey this philosophy to personnel deeply concerned about a patient's welfare.

Patients are basically referred from three sources: (1) inpatient service, (2) outpatient department, (3) self and Community. In addition, an active ward screening program is conducted whereby new admissions are screened on the first day of hospitalization as possible candidates for home care. Age, diagnosis, and functional ability are taken into account and checked before the physician reviews patient and chart and advises in regard to prognosis. Every patient who has been referred is reviewed at a weekly team meeting attended by the physician, nurse, medical social worker, physical therapist, speech therapist, and others. A decision is reached, and the patient, as well as the referring party, is informed of the outcome of the discussion. Typical diagnoses of the patients include the following:

1. diabetes mellitus and its complications, 35 percent;
2. heart disease and strokes, 48 percent;
3. respiratory diseases, 10 percent;
4. cancer, 3 percent;
5. miscellaneous diagnoses, 4 percent.

Types of patients deriving benefit from this program are the following: (1) chronically ill patients, incapacitated to a degree where other care is precluded, who need regularly scheduled monitoring of their treatment and (2) post acutely ill patients in the immediate recovery phase.

There is no time limit for the duration of stay of a patient on our service. Municipal hospitals are unique in that they conduct the only type of home care program wherein the patient can stay on the service for any length of time. Patients with recovery potential can be treated, and patients can be maintained at status quo in the community. The average length of time that these patients are cared for in the program is 6 to 12 months, ranging from 8 to 10 weeks to 5 years or more. Anytime the patient sustains an acute medical episode, he can be readmitted to the parent hospital for intensive care. A home care admission is mandatory, and the home care patient has a bed available to him within the hospital at all times. On occasion the patient may require hospitalization because of a social crisis. The following services are available to patients in their homes: medical, nursing, social service, physical, occupational, and speech therapy; dietary counseling; and laboratory work. In addition the entire range of consultative and diagnostic services within the hospital is at the disposal of the home care patient. If such is needed, the patient is transported to and from the hospital, accompanied by trained escorts. The basic treatment plan, which has been outlined by the physician and the team at the intake conference, can be modified on the spot at any time to suit the patient's need in the environment in which he lives.

The staff psychiatrist sees those patients who present with psychiatric or emotional problems to evaluate the feasibility of maintaining the patient at home without harm to himself or to those around him. He also sees selected patients on an ongoing treatment basis and often helps them to reach decisions that otherwise they would be unable to make. He sees family members and helps them in dealing with the problems of chronic disease and old age. He is always available to all staff members of the home care team to discuss specific problems of handling difficult patients. He acts as a catalyst when temporary or permanent arrangements that are not acceptable to the patient, the family, or the home care staff have to be made, and frequently, guilt feelings are resolved through his intervention. If the medical or social situation becomes such that the patient can no longer be managed adequately at home, institutionalization in a chronic care facility is negotiated and arranged for, if it offers an acceptable solution to patient and family. This provision of psychological and situational support to patient and family and of a judicious medical regimen enables a substantial percentage of the patient population to live out their lives in relative comfort, in the security of their own home.

Summary

Hospital-based home care is a "hospital without walls," a service that provides hospital-type treatment to selected patients in their homes. The entire gamut of professional, paraprofessional, and ancillary care is available to the patient and his family. The services are coordinated by public health nurses stationed in the hospital; they act as a link between the patient and all the services he requires, which are provided inside the hospital, as well as outside by community agencies. Some of the advantages of home care are the following:

1. The patient is more satisfied and is able to function, in however limited a way, in his familiar environment.

2. Professional support of patient and family is provided by supplying the proper service at the time when it is needed.
3. Readmissions to the acute facility are limited by this monitoring of early symptoms of impending crises, both medical and social.
4. Hospital beds are freed for acutely ill patients through earlier discharge of patients back into the community.

Referrals to home care are from: (1) inpatient services, (2) outpatient department, (3) community.

Typical diagnoses of patients on home care: (1) heart disease, (2) strokes, (3) diabetes mellitus, (4) respiratory diseases, (5) cancer, and (6) neuromuscular and skeletal diseases.

Services provided to the patient at home: (1) medical, (2) nursing, (3) social service, (4) physical therapy, (5) speech therapy, (6) dietary counseling, and (7) laboratory work.

With the services provided as outlined, most of these patients can live out their lives at home, in relative comfort and with relative security.

References

Annual Reports, 1968–9, 1970, 1971. Home Care Department, Metropolitan Hospital.

Nauen, R., M. Weitzner, and J. Muller. 1968. "A Method for Planning for Care of Long-Term Patients." *American Journal of Public Health* 58:11, November.

"Self-Evaluation." Home Care Department, Metropolitan Hospital.

Van Dyke, F. and V. Brown. 1968–70. "Home Health Services Study." Columbia University.

Van Dyke, F., V. Brown, and A. M. Thom. 1963. " 'Long Stay' Hospital Care." New York: School of Public Health and Administrative Medicine, Columbia University.

ᎏᎏᎏ 17

Hospice-Based Home Care Services

Mary Kaye Dunn

An outstanding feature of the hospice endeavor, now functioning at Hospice, Inc. (New Haven, Connecticut), is a specialized program of home care service for terminally ill patients. It is anticipated that this service will continue even after a model inpatient facility has been completed. For every 40–44 patients cared for within the projected structure, there would be 100–120 maintained in their own home by the home care staff. The hospice philosophy recognizes that patients do not necessarily "get better" after 5 o'clock or on weekends, and those who are ill may continue to be ill, even around the clock, if they are discharged from the institution. A service must, therefore, be designed to meet varied and complex needs day in and day out.

Such a service must have staff available on a 7-day-a-week, 24-hour-a-day basis, for regularly scheduled visits, as well as for emergency calls. The hospice staff has been organized to support patients and families at any time of the day or night. It has devoted a great deal of energy to maintaining a collaborative relationship with visiting nurse agencies, homemaker and public health nursing agencies, and other health care providers in the community and thus augments the numbers of professionals involved in home care. Every day, visits from hospice, public health, and other agency nurses

153

tend to the needs of patients enrolled in the hospice program; every night, evening nurses follow up on those patients whose needs must be met during these hours.

When the home care program was started at the hospice, the evening shift was introduced on a trial basis. The daytime shift was on duty from 9 A.M. to 5 P.M.; the night shift started at 4 P.M. With this one-hour "overlap" the day staff had time to report to the night staff and alert its members to possible emergencies or problem areas. It soon became evident that many patients needed help at 2 and 3 o'clock in the morning, in a pattern very similar to that of seriously ill hospitalized patients. Personnel were made available to handle emergencies or sudden changes in the course of the patient's condition that occurred after midnight.

On the average, a patient remains under the hospice home care program for approximately three months, a period of time similar to the inpatient hospitalization of a terminal patient in Great Britain. Departing from the British system, which provided the basic model for the hospice ideal in the United States, the home care design of Hospice, Inc., offers more extensive and more structured services and more extended hours during which these are available.

Since March 1974, when the Commissions of Hospitals and Health Care approved the program of Hospice, Inc., until March 1976, approximately 200 patients and their families were served. The hospice philosophy maintains that all services should be family oriented, that the patient should not be isolated from his family. Therefore, the basic unit of care is considered to be the patient and the family. Current systems of reimbursement through private or public health care plans do not, however, ascribe to this concept in making payments. Although an hour spent with a child is, indeed, a service to the parent who is a patient and enables family members to continue to function and cope with what may be a dismal situation, unfortunately current criteria do not regard this as a direct service to the patient.

Obviously, direct care must be addressed to the patient, as well as to the family, but caregiving should be available at the times when the family members are together—even if this occasions visits during the evening hours, when husbands are home from work and children are home from school. This "evening" family is very often different from the "family" seen during the daytime visits. Added to this is the fact that the average age of the patients served by the hospice is 48 years, an age group familiar to those who care for patients with malignant disease.

An integral part of the hospice concept is bereavement followup provided for the patient's family after the patient's death. For the dying patient this has been a great source of comfort, relieving some of the concerns for the welfare of a spouse or children and providing the family with some assurance that visits will be continued and care made available to them on the same level as before their loss to offer the support needed for encouraging the resumption of normal activities in life. The length of time a particular family is followed through the grief process is based on the assessment of that family as individuals with certain specific needs. At the time of the patient's illness the mechanics of the household's functional abilities are assessed, the effectiveness of its individual members is evaluated, and, to some extent, a determination is made concerning just how much help might be needed. On the one-month anniversary of a patient's death either a nurse or a social worker visits a bereaved family. This is an important time for them. For most families, the first 30 days after the death pass quickly because the funeral activities and the immediate period afterwards, with relatives and neighbors visiting, fill many of the hours.

For many, the need for a visit at this time is imperative. It may be difficult for the widow or widower to discuss concerns or feelings when other members of the family are around. Watching mother cry makes children uncomfortable, and mother's open grieving can make it difficult for them, in their own grief, to reach out to provide some support.

Case Report

At the time of the patient's death, a hospice nurse was present. During the patient's illness the wife had expressed the wish to remain with him as much as she possibly could. "I want to be sure he goes out as easy as possible."

Within his last hours she provided the type of ministering care that was very touching, very gentle. In a certain way she was saying, ''I don't want this to happen, but I understand that it is happening.'' She had come to a degree of resolution about the inevitability of her husband's death, and during those last moments she was physically comforting him with touches of her hand and gentle kisses.

On the visit made by the nurse a month later, physical signs of this widow's declining health were observed. The body is a good indicator of how recuperation is taking place on other levels. It was apparent that this woman had not been sleeping. In response to questions about this she said, ''I just cannot sleep at night; that day that he died is such a blur to me.'' Other members of the family were asked what things were like. There was much they had been unable to talk about: it was still too painful. The nurse shared with the woman what she had observed as a person who was present during those last hours. The grieving woman gave a visible sigh of relief and said, ''I am so relieved to know that is what I did those last hours. I have been staying awake at night not able to remember what I had done, and the thought that maybe I wasn't anything I wanted to be for him during those last hours has haunted me.'' The information from the nurse who had actually been there during the final moments of her husband's life provided this woman with the type of comfort that she very much needed at this time.

The research going on at the hospice with regard to the bereavement program has determined that a little bit of intervention at the proper time can often alter a negative situation.

The hospice concept of care for the terminal patient involves attention to the total person, to his physiological, psychological, physical, emotional, and spiritual needs. There are many people who want to sit, talk, and communicate with these patients, but there are not enough people who want to get in and straighten out the sheets or take care of the patient's physical problems. If the patient is uncomfortable or in pain, listening alone will not suffice. In the hierarchy of the patient's needs, perhaps his physical problems should take precedence over the others. The debilitating effects of physical symptoms—physical pain, vomiting, incontinence—impair a person's ability to be integrated within himself and compromise his ability to relate to other people. There is no way to affirm human dignity without the integration of relationships among family members.

What is the nature of our involvement? The hospice tries to provide for anyone who is willing to get into a relationship with a person and be concerned about the others. The hospice strives to help a patient and his family cope with terminal disease. The care that these patients need is often not difficult to provide, if the caregivers observe and listen to determine the specific needs in a specific home. It is an error to assume that care is being provided if existing problems are not identified. It is necessary to ask the patients or family what it is that is needed the most or what it is that they see as the primary problem.

Case Report

A 42-year-old woman with four teenage children wanted to stay at home as long as she possibly could. She was very much in touch with the reality of what was happening to her. On the first assessment visit by the hospice nurse she was found to be in a great deal of pain, vomiting several times during the day, and was quite weakened by having been bedridden. But were these really her problems? She said, "You know, we have a lot of boys in the family [including her husband]; I'm very afraid that they're not going to be able to even manage the household without me." This kind of worry kept her awake at night. The basic maternal instinct of wanting to care for her young was a real focus for her stress. She surprised the nurse by her thought that one was supposed to be in pain if one was dying. The nurse advised her that her physical symptoms could be alleviated in terms of getting the vomiting and nausea under control, as well as achieving control of the pain. Meanwhile, together, they could help the children in the family come to grips with what her greatest concern was: "They don't know how to shop. They don't know how to cook." With the pain and nausea under control, she was able to assume her matriarchal role in the family once again. Though bedridden, she could call out instructions to her boys when they would come home: "What did you get from the grocery store?" "Well, I got five pounds of hamburger." "Well, what you do is you make individual patties." She was back in control of that household, from her bed.

In England there are about 25 to 30 hospices. The medical director of Hospice, Inc., comes from St. Christopher's Hospice in London. An attempt is being made to establish this first hospice in the

United States on the basis of the British model. The physician continues to be involved in the patient's care during the entire course of the illness. Physicians are available to make house calls and provide care to patients at home, particularly when they are no longer able to make it in to an office appointment. Registered nurses, licensed practical nurses, and a full-time social worker run a volunteer program at the hospice that provides professional and lay services, transportation services, volunteer nurses, and shoppers. A certain percentage of time is spent knocking on rectory doors and mobilizing the local priest, minister, or rabbi in whose congregation the patients and family are residing. This very small team from the hospice is able to complement larger agencies and provide services.

One of the most encouraging things about the hospice movement is the momentum that is spreading its concepts around the country, forcing us to review what it is we are doing in our health care system and, perhaps, reorder some of our priorities. The goal of a home care program is not necessarily to have all patients die at home; it happens that about 49 percent of the hospice patients are able to be maintained at home, a figure that is considerably above the national average. But the real goal is to provide appropriate care. Health care professionals are making it clear that the time has come to stop, to think, and to picture some of the problems clearly enough so that we can be agents for change within the existing health care services.

⌘⌘⌘ 18

Hospice Pilot Project in an Acute-Care General Hospital 1975–1976

Sally Woodring

For several years an interdisciplinary group at St. Luke's Hospital in New York City planned a hospice pilot project. The plans were greatly influenced by St. Christopher's Hospice in London and frequent interchanges with its Medical Director, Dr. Cicely Saunders, and other members of the hospice staff. The aim of the concept as it has been adapted to St. Luke's is to improve the care of teminally ill cancer patients within the setting of the acute-care general hospital. The essence of this concept is to enable the patient to live as fully as possible until the moment of death.

It was the feeling of several health professionals that many patients being treated by the present modalities of therapy (i.e., surgery, chemotherapy, radiation, or any combination of these) were in many ways inadequately followed as whole persons. In a hospital that focuses on acute care, the staff often shift their attention from the terminally ill to the acute patient. Two important factors influencing this situation are that the staff is often frustrated by time limitations in relation to all its responsibilities, and very often the staff feels a sense of helplessness in the face of an irreversible disease pro-

159

cess and, at times, a lack of confidence in their ability to approach and cope with the dying patient. As a result, the understanding and caring for the whole patient often occupies a secondary position.

The hospice team at St. Luke's Hospital is composed of one full-time nurse clinical specialist who acts as coordinator of the project. The other team members are part time: one surgeon (medical director), one psychiatrist, two nurse clinical specialists, one social worker, and one chaplain. The team follows terminally ill cancer patients with a three- to six-month prognosis from nine general medical-surgical floors. While the patient is in the hospital, the hospice team members visit him frequently, each member using his special expertise and personality in meeting the patient's needs. The first concern is with symptom control, since a person cannot concentrate on interactions with staff or family while suffering physically. Rapport is gradually developed between the patient and team, as well as among team, staff, and family. Since the hospice is a consultative service, much attention is given to the support and education of the hospital staff to enable it to provide the necessary individualized care of these patients. During the inpatient period, usually one hospice team member becomes the primary member involved with a particular patient. This relationship provides more understanding and support, since the patient feels a personal attachment to one person. With the knowledge that this relationship will continue after the patient returns home and that the hospice team will facilitate readmission to the hospital when necessary, the patient and family are often more willing to make arrangements for the patient's discharge, even if it is for only a brief time.

Plans for the patient's return home are made by discussions among the patient and family members, the hospice team, home care, and the floor staff. During these planning sessions, decisions are made about what kind of home support is needed, and appropriate agencies are contacted. Sometimes a visiting nurse will visit the patient once a week, a home health aide will be with the patient four to eight hours a day, or 24 hours if needed, or the family will simply be reassured of support when needed if they can care for the patient themselves. The key idea is individualized care; each patient and family unit is evaluated individually and continues to be evaluated so that the plan of care can be updated as the patient's condition changes. The patient and family are given the hospice team's names and phone numbers so that they can reach the team whenever the need arises.

Several means of support to the outpatient have been developed by the team: (1) A team member sees the patient during his scheduled clinic appointments to reassess the situation and act as a liaison between the patient and clinic doctor and nurses. (2) If the patient needs medication before a scheduled clinic appointment, the hospice physician will write a prescription, and the hospice nurse will get it filled and plan to meet the family member or attendant sent to pick up the medication. This saves the patient an unnecessary trip to the hospital. (3) If the patient needs to see a physician before a scheduled appointment, he can see the hospice physician in the emergency room within 24 hours of his request. A hospice nurse and/or other hospice team member also confers with the physician and patient in the emergency room to assess the situation further, continue emotional support, and act as a patient advocate in conserving the patient's energy by helping him avoid long waiting periods for physicians or medications. (4) Sometimes problems that arise at home can be solved simply by the family's or patient's calling the hospice and receiving advice by phone. (5) Most of the hospice patients live in the St. Luke's catchment area, so that the team members can easily make home visits when necessary to evaluate physical problems or to offer emotional support to the patient and family.

When the patient needs assistance in traveling to the clinic, arrangements are made for an ambulette to transport the patient to and from the hospital. Occasionally, since many of the patients are from the lower socioeconomic population, the hospice's special funds provide taxi fare for patients who otherwise would have to suffer the torments of public transportation when they are feeling very sick. Since St. Luke's Hospital serves a heterogeneous population where many families live in substandard housing and have inadequate finances, much support is needed if the family is to care for the patient at home. Coordination between the hospice, home care, visiting nurse service, and other agencies is crucial in this situation.

Within a week of a patient's death, the hospice team member

who has become closest to the patient contacts the family and invites them to visit or talk by phone. If the family wishes counseling about funeral arrangements, this is provided. This team member calls the family again in four to six weeks and offers to meet with them. If there seem to be abnormal mourning or family disturbances, the team member consults with the team and may refer the family for further counseling. Contact with the family is maintained through the first year of bereavement. There are plans to initiate an ongoing bereavement group, led by the team psychiatrist and social worker, in which family members can interact with other bereaved people on a weekly basis for three months. It is hoped that this will provide bereaved families with more support and perspective regarding their loss. Again, at the end of these three months, the group leaders will evaluate each family member and make appropriate referrals for more therapy if this seems needed.

Case Studies

During its first 10 months, the St. Luke's Hospice program enabled two patients to die at home as they wished. One was H. M., a 53-year-old woman with cancer of the lung, metastasized to the breast, liver, and brain. While receiving radiation therapy in the hospital, she suffered much nausea and vomiting, and her only wish was to go home. The one thing she requested to make her hospital admission more tolerable was to have her poodle visit her. Since the hospice allows patients to see their pets, this was arranged and resulted in a great increase of morale in the patient and among the hospital staff. Knowing that the patient, who lived alone, would need a lot of bedside care, the social worker arranged for H. M.'s friend, who lived in her building, to move into H. M.'s apartment. Her friend acted as an attendant and was reimbursed by Medicaid. The hospice nurse visited the patient at home a number of times to bring pain medication, to assess her physical condition and determine if a clinic appointment was necessary, and to offer emotional support both to H. M. and her friend. Twice the patient was transported by ambulette to the emergency room, where the hospice physician examined her and altered her medication regimen. As the end drew near, the hospice nurse and chaplain talked with H. M. to make certain that she still wished to remain at home. They also counseled H. M.'s friend and discussed what she planned when H. M. died and what funeral arrangements would be made. The hospice nurse talked with the friend a number of times after H. M.'s death and found a part-time housekeeping job for her. Even though H. M.'s apartment was very modest and in a poor neighborhood, it was "home" to her, where she wished to end her days surrounded by things familiar to her, including her dog and her friend. Hospice's intervention in terms of pain and nausea control and emotional support to H. M. and her friend seemed to make the difference in enabling this patient to die the way she chose.

The second case of a patient's dying at home was A. H., a 55-year-old woman with cancer of the pancreas, metastasized to the stomach and liver. When she first went to St. Luke's Hospital in the spring of 1975, she was a belligerent, demanding person complaining of much pain. Hospice's first goal in October 1975 when picking up the patient was to control this pain by using oral methadone at regular intervals around the clock. The methadone was gradually increased and Phenergan was added to the regimen. Although the patient lost much weight and lived in a small, dark room in a welfare hotel, her will to live was strong once the pain was controlled. She complained of feeling weak and "not wanting to be drowsy the rest of my life," and so prednisone and Ritalin were added to her medication, resulting in an increased appetite and more energy.

Hospice knew her as an inpatient only seven days. During the final three months of her life, A. H. was seen every one to two weeks in the emergency room by the hospice physician to assess her physical condition. The hospice nurse, chaplain, and social worker also saw her during these appointments to make sure that she understood her medication schedule, to assist her in obtaining her welfare checks, and to offer emotional support. When there was some question of her emotional status, it was arranged for the hospice psychiatrist to interview her with the rest of the team present. She was reassured that there was a group of concerned people coordinating their plan of care for her. Eventually she complained that she was too weak and the weather was too cold for her to come to the clinic. One of her two welfare hotel friends, who by this time were providing 24-hour-a-day care, picked up her medication from the hospice nurse as needed.

During her last month, the chaplain and three hospice nurses visited A. H. a number of times at home—to bring her food and medication, to catheterize her, to offer support to her friends, and to talk about her past life, present illness, thoughts about life after death, her feelings of lack of faith, and whatever else was on her mind. The patient, although extremely weak and requiring large amounts of pain medicine, continued her interest in conversation and in the lives of others. She and one hospice nurse shared an interest in music. This resulted in that nurse's bringing her 11-member madrigal group to the patient's room to sing for 20 minutes. This event proved to be enormously significant for both A. H. and her friend, both of whom dressed especially for the occasion and talked about it at length afterward.

The patient's condition deteriorated rapidly, and she gradually became less responsive. During her last six days, the chaplain and two hospice nurses visited her every one to two days. The day A. H. died, the friend talked for a long time with the one hospice nurse who was especially close to A. H. The friend expressed her feelings of the past week and plans for the next few days. Since the patient had made no specific requests for a funeral, the hospice chaplain offered to conduct a memorial service at the St. Luke's Hospital Chapel for the two hotel friends, several friends from A. H.'s job, and the hospice team. This seemed to be an appropriate means of closure for all. The hospice nurses have been in contact with the one hotel friend several times by telephone and visit since the memorial service.

In both cases, the coordinated efforts of the hospice team, social service, and home care made it possible for a terminally ill cancer patient to die at home, surrounded by those things most meaningful to her. The patients were kept as comfortable as possible while remaining alert enough to continue some measure of "living" to the end.

In summary, the St. Luke's Hospice is a unique program adapting the hospice concept to an acute-care general hospital. As such, the hospice is helping to demonstrate that curing is not the only kind of therapy to be received in a hospital. "Curing the mind" can be another proof of one's being a successful practitioner. The St. Luke's Hospice is a model that others can adapt to their particular hospitals, which may have different problems and strengths. The hospice approach expands our humanity in treating patients as people rather than as disease entities.

AUTHOR'S NOTE: *Since 1976, there have been changes in personnel and direction of this hospice program. During this period, 300 patients have been cared for.*

⚛⚛⚛ 19

Problems and Considerations for Effective Home Care of the Cancer Patient

Kenneth Lefebvre

It is becoming more common for cancer patients to receive chemotherapy either as the primary mode of treatment or as an adjunct to radiotherapy or surgery. Some of these patients are receiving immunotherapy, others are getting the treatment prophylactically, but most have been referred to the chemotherapist because their disease has been unresponsive to other forms of treatment or because chemotherapy is the treatment of choice.

The author has been involved in the psychosocial component of a medical oncology service. The goal of this service was to provide more adequate medical care by being aware of factors, other than physical considerations, that can influence a patient's ability to tolerate both the treatment and the diagnosis of cancer. Home care has become an important issue, since many patients have to be hospitalized only during the first course of therapy to monitor side effects and when complications of the therapy or the disease process demand it.

On the patient's first visit to the outpatient clinic, an interview is conducted by both the staff psychologist and social worker. Using a structured interview designed for this purpose, they assess how the disease has affected the patient's life, what the reactions of family and friends are, what the patient has been told about his disease, and what the patient expects from the therapy.

New patients are discussed at a weekly meeting attended by physicians, the oncology nurse, the social worker, the psychologist, and laboratory personnel. The goals of this meeting are to provide all physicians on the service with some information about each new patient and to attempt to identify patients and/or families who will have a difficult time adjusting to the disease.

This chapter deals with some of the problems of patients who are receiving chemotherapy for palliative care. Three areas are especially important for coordinated and appropriate home care. A major concern for any noncurable cancer patient is the terminal nature of his disease. Although great strides have been made in the treatment of cancer, the diagnosis still means death to many people, and so the patient is often acutely aware of the serious nature of his disease.

However, this awareness is affected by the fact that many patients who have not responded well to other treatments often have good initial response to anticancer drugs. For example, a patient's palpable tumor mass may shrink in size, and nuclear scans may show decreased neoplastic activity. While this is certainly a good sign, the results may be only temporary. Yet patients will feel as though they have been given a reprieve from certain death. The problems arise when the patient and family members have to deal with the reality of the drugs' becoming less effective and the cancer's becoming more widespread.

Such a situation emphasizes that cancer care cannot be only physical. An approach considering psychosocial factors and resources is most important with any chronic illness. This is especially true when both the patient and family members have to adjust to many changes caused by the disease. The author has been involved in a study assessing such changes, and preliminary results indicate that such basic activities as eating, sleep, and sexual and recreational activities are all disturbed. Communication patterns, conceptions of disease and suffering, and opinions about the quantity versus quality of life are all critical factors in an approach stressing total patient care.

A fundamental problem is partially semantic. What does the word *terminal* mean? Many patients hearing the diagnosis *cancer* feel they have a terminal disease. Physicians may have similar feelings but do not consider a person terminal until the patient's performance level is so impaired that intensive supportive care either at home or in the hospital is required. The difference is one of emphasis. The patient may feel that he is terminal because life as he knows it (without the label "cancer patient" or the stresses of chemotherapy) has come to an end. The patient's view is behavioral and personal, the physician's, physical.

Given these two points of view, it is easy to see how communications can get garbled. For example, a physician's obvious pleasure at a decreased tumor size can be misinterpreted by anxious patients or family members to mean that the patient will be "cured." Naturally, no one wants to remind a patient or family member continually that the good response may only be temporary. But sometimes the staff's silence can be taken as support for unrealistic and overly optimistic expectations for treatments.

Patients often realize that they are becoming more ill but try to deny this fact and minimize disability by acting "as if" they can continue to do the things they've always done. When a patient is thwarted in these attempts, he may direct his feelings of anger and frustration toward family members or members of the medical team.

At this point it is vital to help the patient accept and adjust to decreased productivity and altered self-image. This adjustment is complicated, for other family members feel the need to do something, to be helpful in some way, to draw themselves into the patient's life. There are cases in which family members who have not been close for many years are drawn together during these times. These may include former spouses, married children with their own families, in-laws, siblings, and relations by marriage. Attempts to be helpful on these persons' parts quite often backfire and put additional stress on the patient and his immediate family.

Many extended family members are torn between obligations to their own families and to the patient. Because they feel some responsibility to help but may be overextended or not very capable of dealing with stress themselves, it is easy to see how the end result can be confusion and distress.

Physicians, nurses, and other members of the health care team get calls from many different family members reporting accurate, distorted, or bizarre accounts of a patient's behavior. In one case a patient's second wife reported her husband was drinking heavily, was constantly depressed, and was threatening suicide. The patient reported that his wife was very anxious and was unable to deal with his cancer. This situation intensified and was resolved when the patient returned to his first wife. Paradoxically, the patient had reported that he had divorced this woman because he didn't want her "to get anything when I die."

Such an example illustrates the complex problems that can arise in families. It is often nonproductive to spend time trying to find out what is "really happening." It is more important to realize that such behavior is characteristic of a family system under stress. Different medical staff receive conflicting information and, therefore, it is easy to conceptualize the problem differently and to identify different persons as "the problem." We have found that a better approach is to set up a family meeting in which the medical staff, including doctors, nurses, the social worker, and psychologist, can meet with family members and discuss the implications of the disease and offer possible alternatives to help the whole family cope with a difficult problem.

A regular function of the psychosocial team is consultation with the inpatient nursing staff of the oncology service. It is often difficult to understand the actions of family members without knowing some of the patient's social history and the role that he or she plays and had played within the family. Weekly staff conferences focus on such issues and provide a setting in which staff can talk privately about patients or families that irritate or confuse them. These meetings also allow staff to consider different ways of interacting with patients or families. Cancer nursing can often be very frustrating because at times it demands that staff not do anything, at least in terms of traditional nursing skills. Often the most that a nurse can do is sit with a patient, hold his hand, and try to share his fears and concerns. Empathy for the personal reactions of family members—no matter how emotional or disruptive to floor routine—is a valuable and important factor in providing total patient care.

The goal of palliative care is not to cure but to minimize the pain and suffering associated with any chronic or terminal disease. The social system of hospital–family–patient is important and must be considered in planning such care.

There is a tendency for cancer patients to endow their physicians, especially cancer specialists, with godlike qualities and powers. This can lead to many problems if the patient begins to bring every medical problem to the oncologist rather than maintain liaison with his primary physician. While it is flattering to be told that "only you can help," it does not make for good medical care.

The medical oncology service has found the following factors to be important in providing coordinated patient care:

1. Stress the importance for the patient to maintain contact with his primary physician, as well as with other consulting specialists.
2. Assess the kinds of medical facilities necessary for the patient's potential needs and help with facilitating or initiating referrals to agencies such as skilled nursing homes and home nursing care agencies.
3. Consider the ability of the family to deal with the stresses of a home-bound patient and in some cases recognize a family's inability to cope with such a situation.
4. Determine the patient's preferences about his own medical care and his feelings of how the disease has affected the family.
5. Identify and help, if possible, with problems that may be too painful for the family to broach. For example, it has been necessary several times to help patients write wills or make funeral arrangements. Such issues are sometimes too difficult for family members to raise, but they need to be confronted lest they produce additional difficulties after the death of the patient.
6. Reassure the patient that his local hospital and physician will be able to treat his symptoms of pain and discomfort and that the patient can often be as comfortable at home as in the hospital.
7. Inform the patient and family as fully as possible about what symptoms to expect as the disease progresses. This can reduce a family's anxiety by

removing some fear of the unknown and prevent a family from rushing the patient to the hospital every time a progressive symptom manifests itself.

If anything has impressed the psychosocial component of the medical oncology service, it is the need for coordinated discharge planning, sometimes beginning at the point the patient is referred to the chemotherapist. Discharge planning means much more than simply giving a patient a date when he can leave the hospital. To do effective discharge planning with any patient, three important factors must be considered:

1. The problem of personal reactions to rapidly changing medical conditions or long-term hospitalization is the first factor. Early assessment of the ability of the patient and family to deal with the stresses of cancer is achieved by routinely discussing new referrals and attempting to identify those persons needing counseling or close attention. Additional patient and family interviews are helpful in identifying families that may need supplemental medical, psychological, social, or rehabilitative services. Such work needs to be started early because it is easy to delay intervention until a crisis situation mandates it. Such delay can, however, make any intervention less effective because the interim coping styles and mechanisms become more rigid and therefore less amenable to change.

2. The lack of communication and coordination between inpatient staff, outpatient staff, and the family is the second factor. During the course of the disease, the patient may require a number of hospitalizations, as well as many diagnostic tests and special nuclear scans. If there is poor communication between both staffs and the family, certain problems are likely to occur: (a) Patients may arrive at the outpatient clinic and be told that they have no appointment for the day. Patients often think that inpatient staff make outpatient appointments, while the physician is under the impression that the patient knew all along that this was the patient's responsibility. The lesson learned is that it is impossible to be too explicit when acquainting patients with new medical routines. Time should also be spent in determining if the patient really understood what different people on the staff were trying to say. We often do not communicate as clearly as we think we do. (b) Oncology floor nurses can become frustrated and irritated when patients with whom they are not familiar are admitted for long-term care on a unit that was specifically identified as providing short-term, acute care and inpatient chemotherapy. If such patients have

to be admitted because of extenuating circumstances or because they are undergoing a special procedure, this should be clearly explained to the floor staff. A little explanation can make both patient and staff more comfortable. (c) A patient may arrive expecting treatment and then be told that he must return at a later date because reports of diagnostic tests are not available. Patient charts should be reviewed before the appointment, and if such a problem is anticipated, the patient can be contacted by phone and rescheduled to avoid a wasted trip. (d) Family members become confused when several medical specialists answer their questions slightly differently. For example, one physician might tell a patient that it is important that he stay in the hospital for a liver scan, while a colleague will say such procedures could be delayed for a month. Although differences of opinion are to be expected in any professional discipline, it is important to resolve those differences beyond the earshot of the family and patient.

3. Crisis-oriented problem solving that results only in perpetuating a crisis situation is the third factor. Whereas it is often inappropriate and unnecessary to reiterate to a patient that he may only have a year or two to live, it is equally inappropriate for staff members to delay making contingency plans for the patient's eventual deteriorated medical condition. This is certainly one case in which waiting to cross the bridge when you get to it may require rebuilding the bridge first. Nonmedical personnel, like social workers and psychologists, can be quite helpful in assessing and identifying problem areas, as well as in facilitating services such as home health care, medical supplies, and nursing home referrals.

Close liaison among all members of a health care delivery team can result in comprehensive and coordinated patient care with a minimum of frustrations for all involved.

Acknowledgment

This project was made possible through a fellowship awarded by the East Tennessee Cancer Research Center and by the professional support of Drs. Stephen Krauss, Tony Girardi, and Leonard Handler.

≋≋≋ 20

Patient Counseling in Home Care

Richard Chassé

The vantage point provided to the patient counselor by the rehabilitation and continuing care project at the Medical College of Virginia (MCV) is that of giving him the opportunity to observe the family in its "home atmosphere." In many instances a visit to the home provides the counselor with a broader and a more in-depth picture of the reality with which a patient contends outside the hospital. The hospital at best provides a somewhat artificial atmosphere for the patient. It is an accepted fact that most patients regress emotionally in the strange hospital surroundings and are often called upon by the physician and staff to surrender their personal authority. An immediate result is that the patient undergoes treatment submissively while repressing anger, helplessness, and limitation of self-expression. Often, the patient's inner ability to choose and express what he feels is right for him becomes dysfunctional. It is in this state that a patient is now judged to be unable to cope with his or her disease.

In such a hospital atmosphere another professional may be seen as just another body invading not only "my" personal space but also "my" inner space. The intervention of such a person may cause

This project was supported by NCI Contract No. 1-CN-45144.

some reticence on the part of the patient. During the hospital stay the patient will either submit to this intervention or present a picture of self-sufficiency. Either way the patient will attempt to maintain his personal identity and independence.

Upon his release from the hospital, the patient, more often than not, is able to regain most, if not all, of his precious personal authority. He knows his own turf, and the disease and aftermath of a serious illness may have changed to some degree his ability to cope with what may have been a livable situation before his illness. It is not long before the feeling of helplessness returns and decreases the patient's ability to cope even at home.

Essentially in the hospital the patient's setting has been, at best, artificial. Whether counseling is done at the bedside or in the counselor's private office, the hospital situation is viewed by the patient as a temporary change. At home the change is encountered as a change in reality, and the changes can no longer be overlooked or denied. Often patients will at this point wonder if they will ever regain their self-confidence and self-determination. This is the time when a home visit by the hospital patient counselor has proven to be an added asset to the patient and his health care. It is also the time when the counselor is able to see firsthand the realities with which the patient has to contend. In addition to actually observing the environment of the patient, the counselor is able to maintain and create a new link in the relationship with the patient. During the home visit the patient can be observed in his natural habitat, and his strengths and weaknesses can be more readily seen within the context of the whole family. Usually the family dynamics, which are normally interrupted during the hospitalization, are resumed at a near normal level. It is within this context that the patient's continuing health care and maintenance of a high quality of life will occur.

It seems rather obvious that family therapy is needed in a health care situation. A crisis has arisen in the family, which has strained or destroyed whatever coping mechanisms may have been available in the past. It is also the time when intervention by a professional is needed but most likely is least available. If the family is aware of its need, it may not be able to answer that need for help, because the patient must leave his own turf and return to the artificial atmosphere of the practitioner's office to solve a problem that exists "back there." To my knowledge there are very few, if any, professionals who will actually consent to providing individual or family therapy in the home. The primary reason, I fear, is that going into the home is a rather inefficient manner in which to conduct the business of providing help. I must confess I also believe it is a very inefficient use of the professional's time and skill if we consider it in terms of dollars and cents. In fact the professional's ability to be of service to his patients is cut at least in half. If the professional has an eight-hour workday and sees clients at the rate of one per hour, he can see eight people on a given day. However, if he sees the patient in the home, he must provide the minimum of two hours per patient. His patient load is cut in half, and in order for him to maintain his standard of living he must increase his fee for the home visit. A vicious circle begins with no one benefiting. The patient cannot financially afford the visit, nor can the counselor. In addition, the four "other" potential patients simply cannot be seen.

This presents a strong argument, perhaps the strongest, against the home visit. However, we are not dealing with efficiency but with quality. When the cancer rehabilitation and continuing care project was conceived at MCV, I was given the opportunity to be a patient counselor on the project with the express mission of conducting home visits with the patients. At first the caseload and other responsibilities were quite manageable, and I soon discovered the value of meeting the patient and his family on their "home turf." I felt very much like a guest in the home, especially if my first contact was made in the home by a referral from our staff. In one sense this was a roadblock to therapy, but in another sense it strengthened the patient's and family's ability to assume their rightful authority over what was happening to them.

However, it was not long before the patient load and project responsibilities increased and conflicted. The staff began to seek me out to consult with them on what might be happening with a given patient emotionally. I soon found myself dealing with patients, families, staff, and the intimate relationships that arose from these interactions. I became a traffic cop in the arena of feelings and the provision of the staff's emotional support.

What are the alternatives? More effective use of my time soon became the following: stop in-hospital activity, stop home visiting, increase the number of patient counselors, train the staff to deal with basic emotional supportive care, train volunteers, make more referrals, and so on. None of the solutions were adequate or feasible.

Owing to my ministerial background a verse of scripture would often come to mind and eventually to my lips: "The poor you will always have with you." I substituted the word *sick* for *poor*, although at MCV they often become synonymous. I realized that somehow a compromise of all the solutions mentioned was needed. I settled on the compromise of seeing the patients who exhibited the greatest emotional need both in the home and in the hospital clinics and leaving the less critical situations to the staff members, who after a year's experience were beginning to provide excellent emotional support at a different level. I also compromised by combining home visits and office visits for several reasons. I discovered that if I dealt with patients solely in my office by appointment, they would often miss the appointment because of financial problems, transportation problems, and sometimes because of physical status. As a result of missed appointments patients could conceivably not be seen for a month or longer, and the effectiveness of therapy quickly diminished.

On the other hand, making frequent home visits often produced some diminishing returns for the patient. I mentioned that initially I was treated as a guest in the home for one or two visits. After several visits another reaction occurred. I became an invader of privacy in "the refuge" (their home) from the hospital. Needless to say, this was intensified by the area of my profession. Realizing this, I began to experiment by alternating office visits and home visits. I was soon able to increase my home visitations and was then able to maintain a higher level of therapy with the patient. The immediate result of this alternative was twofold: I was able to observe and maintain contact with the family's environment, and the patient and the family were better able to discern my role and more clearly define how they could use my expertise. In short, we became more comfortable with each other.

By using this third method of alternating visits, an ideal of my ministry and profession was better realized. I call this ideal reconciliation. By moving in two worlds, that of the hospital and of the home, the patient and I were able to bring together two real yet seemingly distinct realities. The artificiality of the hospital, which fragmented the patient's world, and the unknown environs of the home for the counselor were merged to create a continuum of experience for the patient and the counselor.

Translated in terms of quality of life, the family and patient are able to put together their fragmented experience by relating, not to separate circumstances, but to a singular experience of a person involved in the reality of total health care. Patient and family are able to converse more freely about their hospital and home experience knowing that I am able to share both areas of concern with them.

Another innovative aspect of our project has been the expansion of the various professional roles involved. This has occurred by design and by necessity. Everyone on the project, from physician to secretary, has not only become aware of the existence of another professional treating the patient and the family but also knowledgeable about the capabilities and expertise of his fellow professionals. From my viewpoint my contribution to our team has been that of providing consultation and education to the staff members in the areas of emotional and religious reactions to serious debilitating illness such as cancer.

It is difficult for any service-oriented professional to avoid encountering these two areas of involvement while working with a patient and his family. In the hospital the professional may always appear rushed when unavoidably called out of the patient's room to answer a call on the paging system. In the home, however, these escapes are not readily available, and the patient has the sense that he is the only one being visited. Therefore, the home provides the setting for asking some of those unanswered questions that invariably linger and demand an answer. Nor is the practitioner able to escape very easily. As a result, the practitioner has needed to develop some expertise in communication and supportive care.

Often the visiting practitioner is seen and expected to be the counselor or advice-giver to the patient and family. During team conferences consultation is readily available. However, it is often necessary in the day-to-day routine for various staff members to seek an on-the-spot consultation before or after making a home visit. During these informal consultations two things occur: the patient's situation is discussed, and some decisions and plans are made. This is not very different from what occurs in many areas of the hospital. What is different, however, is that I often ask what the staff member feels about the patient. It is essential that the practitioner know what he feels about his patient in order to treat the patient comprehensively. When the project first started, members of the staff approached me for books to read and even for a course on what to say when a patient would ask such and such. My reply was often "No book or course can teach that. Let the patient teach you."

Through the consultation, the staff has come to feel comfortable in working with our patients. Many have acquired basic skills that psychology graduates have yet to learn. As a direct result, moreover, referrals have not been as necessary as in the beginning of the project, and what referrals we do have and make are of a higher quality, demanding more professional expertise. At the same time there is less demand for outside supportive care on the part of the patient or family because they have been able to rely on the various staff members who are truly active listeners.

Along with the improved supportive care of the patient, the staff have been able to more realistically and effectively establish goals with the patient and the family in their health care. Staff members have dealt more objectively with the families because they are better able to deal with their own subjective feelings. The direct result of this expanded role has been to provide better objective health care planning, sensitively agreed upon with the family and patient. The quality of life, which has been elusive to measure, has become more tangible in that the lives of the patient are not merely tolerable but truly more livable.

⩘⩘⩘ 21

Senior Companion Program

Marie G. Wilson and Regina Sugrue

The senior companion program (SCP) in New York City was funded in July 1974 by ACTION—the Federal volunteer agency—as one of 18 demonstration projects in the country. United Neighborhood Houses (UNH), a federation of settlement houses, sponsored the program in New York and operates the senior companion program in 13 neighborhood-based settlement houses in Manhattan, Bronx, Brooklyn, and Queens.

The program has two major goals: to provide meaningful community service roles for low-income people 60 years and older and pay them a small stipend and to provide companionship and services to isolated or homebound older adults in their own homes.

The intent of the program is to develop a person-to-person relationship between the visiting senior companion and homebound or isolated client and, through this relationship, to assist people in living in their own homes and in participating in their communities, and to prevent unnecessary or premature institutionalization. The activities in which clients and senior companions engage flow from the relationship and depend on the needs of the clients and the skills of the senior companions. These include reading, talking, crafts, escort to clinics and senior centers, and linkage to other services. If clients are

178

hospitalized, visits continue at the hospital and resume at home upon discharge.

Seventy-three adults were recruited, participated in a 40-hour orientation, and visit the same two people each day, five days a week for two hours a day. In addition to the stipend, senior companions, who serve 20 hours a week, receive transportation reimbursement, a meal a day, insurance coverage, and an annual medical examination. A project director coordinates the citywide program, and at each settlement house there is an on-site supervisor. Senior companions receive monthly in-service training at UNH to acquire additional skills. There are also semimonthly group meetings at each site for the senior companions, as well as individual sessions to discuss each senior companion's service and to assist with the individual needs of both senior companions and clients.

Clients are served in the target areas of each of the 13 settlement houses. They are referred to the program by social service agencies, families, hospitals, nutrition programs, and others or are self-referred. Most of the people live alone, with few if any relatives or friends nearby.

Before a client is accepted, an application form is completed detailing the needs of the person, as well as the kinds of short- or long-term services required. In addition, clients sign a letter authorizing the SCP to provide service. A visit to the client's home is made by the supervisor before assignment of a senior companion to explain the program. The supervisor also accompanies the senior companion on the first visit. For the majority of persons served by the senior companion program, it becomes the primary agency responding to their needs. For example, in addition to the daily visit and activities with the senior companion, the program assists persons in obtaining other necessary services, such as homemaking assistance, medical attention, legal assistance, or entitlements such as SSI, rent exemption, and half-fare cards. The vital linkage to other social or governmental agencies is provided by the senior companions, on-site supervisors, and the project director at UNH.

From November 1974 to March 1976, 16 clients have died, and currently eight senior companions are working with terminally ill patients. Of this number, some of the clients were or are aware their illness is terminal. In all instances, the senior companions have been aware of the diagnosis. In one situation the doctor discussed the illness with the senior companion, but not the client. It is our opinion that, in each of these instances, senior companions help to bring comfort, dignity, and hope to their dying clients. In some situations they were also of assistance to families. For the majority of senior companions this is not the first experience with a dying person. Senior companions range in age from 60 to 86 years. Often their younger years were spent in other countries or the rural United States, and their generation dealt more comfortably with a person dying at home. They can and do bring a layperson's life experience with death to the program, an experience missing from the past lives of younger people—lay or professional.

The kinds of interactions between senior companions and terminally ill clients have varied, depending on the personalities and realities, such as whether the client acknowledges awareness of his/her illness. Some examples will illustrate the various kinds of interactions and relationships that developed between the senior companion and the client.

Example 1: Mary McC., a 69-year-old woman, was assigned to visit Charlotte F, 88 years old, in the spring of 1975. Charlotte's husband had died 15 years before. There were no surviving relatives and no children. The situation was referred to us by a hospital's social services department, which discovered that Charlotte was living alone, not eating, and required hospitalization for a diagnostic workup. Charlotte had been refusing hospitalization because she was concerned about her apartment in an otherwise abandoned building. Mary, the senior companion, was assigned and within a few weeks gained the confidence of Charlotte—enough so that Charlotte entered the hospital, where a tentative diagnosis of a terminal illness was made. In addition to daily visits to the hospital, Mary also watered the plants, picked up the mail, and so on. Charlotte wanted to be discharged. It was not considered feasible for her to return to the abandoned building. Therefore, the Senior Companion supervisor found her a room in a nearby hotel. She was discharged, and Mary's visits continued at "home." Although social workers and visiting nurses were involved, Charlotte discussed her situation only with Mary. Charlotte knew she was going to die. The two women talked about the past, as well as the future. Both looked forward to Thanksgiving lunch at the settlement house. Charlotte once told Mary that plans for her funeral had to be made, and both women picked out clothing and made arrangements for a funeral. Charlotte had to reenter the hospital one month before she died in January 1976; Mary visited her daily. She remained lucid until she died. The funeral was attended by Mary and her supervisor and was in accordance with Charlotte's wishes.

Example 2: Ben C., a 67-year-old senior companion, was assigned to Mr. P., a 94-year-old man in December 1974. Mr. P. was blind and frail, but otherwise healthy, physically and mentally. He lived in a Housing Authority project on the Lower East Side. His surviving children were older than the senior companion and lived in other parts of the city. Ben and Mr. P. belonged to different racial and religious groups. After visiting for several months, suddenly one Monday morning, Ben arrived to find Mr. P. incontinent and hallucinating. Mr. P.'s 75-year-old daughter was distraught and immobilized. Ben called an ambulance, and Mr. P. was rushed to the hospital, where kidney failure was diagnosed. Further testing showed prostate cancer. The doctors wanted to operate, and the family refused. Mr. P. regained his lucidity after dialysis treatment, and he too refused the operation. He remained in intensive care connected to life-maintaining machinery. Ben was able to convince the hospital staff to allow him to visit daily in the intensive care unit. He and Mr. P. talked; Mr. P. was not afraid of dying. He said that, at 94 years, he was ready, but he was angered at his helpless state. Ben helped him deal with his anger. They talked about his life, his accomplishments, and his readiness to meet his God. Gradually, they talked less, and Ben would sit at the bedside, holding Mr. P.'s hand or otherwise indicating his presence, ready to respond if Mr. P. wanted anything. Ben also would comfort the son and daughter, both in their 70s, whose grief made them unable to respond to their father. Mr. P. died four weeks after hospitalization. Ben cried but assured a concerned project director that, while he was naturally upset because he liked Mr. P., mostly he felt good at being able to help him. Ben hoped that in a similar situation somebody would do the same for him. Within a week, he accepted another assignment.

Example 3: Frieda S. was assigned to Mr. M., a married man in his late 50s, with a terminal illness that restricted his mobility. His grown children lived elsewhere, and his wife had to work to help support the family, leaving Mr. M. alone during the day. Frieda was reluctant to accept the assignment because she felt there was nothing she could do. We explained to her that her cheerful, extrovert personality might help Mr. M. live as fully as possible as long as possible. She agreed to try. At first, Mr. M. met Frieda at the door of his apartment looking unkempt and in his bathrobe. Now he greets her dressed in trousers, shirt, and shoes. He will not talk about his illness, but they watch TV together, eat lunch, discuss current events and their children, joke, and talk about dancing at Roseland sometime soon. Frieda is delighted at her success, Mrs. M. is able to continue working, and Mr. M. feels he has a pleasant, viable present and a future.

Example 4: Theresa G. was assigned to Miss D., a 78-year-old woman one year ago. Miss D. lived with her aged mother, her only relative, whose heart was failing, and we hoped to help Miss D. deal with the increasing frailty of her mother, as well as herself. One day Miss D. confided to the senior companion that she felt a lump in her breast, but her fears prevented her going to a doctor. Theresa herself has cancer in remission and helped convince the client to seek medical attention. The tumor was cancerous and had metastasized. Miss D. is receiving outpatient therapy, leaving her nauseous and weak. The doctor refused to discuss the illness with the patient or the mother and instead discussed it with Theresa but forbade her to discuss this with the client. Theresa, who had had chemotherapy herself, is able to discuss treatment with the client, empathizing with the feeling and reassuring her that what she experiences will pass. In addition, she is able to assist in helping the client's mother and thereby relieve another source of anxiety for Miss D.

In these examples, senior companions, as lay persons who are not family members, have been able to provide help to terminally ill people in their own homes and/or hospitals. Their help is not medical or professional. They do not reject the dying but help prevent human isolation at the end of a life and bring comfort, hope, and dignity to their clients. The senior companions were asked to discuss their feelings about working with clients who have a terminal illness. With one exception, all senior companions said they would do it again, even though they were all saddened by the loss of the person they served. They feel that they were helpful, that they performed a service no one else, not the doctor, or social worker, or family, provided. All feared they would not be able to be so helped if they became terminally ill, and this concern—dying alone with no one to talk with or no one to know—seemed to be a more overwhelming fear than the fear of death itself. Some noted that they indeed felt less afraid of dying since their recent, close connection with a terminally ill person. One woman, speaking for others, said that she felt she got to know herself better, to put her own life in some perspective.

In the senior companion program, the staff has had to deal with the issue of close identification between the senior companon and the client who is an age peer in frailer, more isolated circumstances. The staff has found that allowing the issue to be discussed openly, listening and responding to the feelings generated, and using a developmental theoretical approach to aging are of assistance. The 40-hour orientation; monthly, group-oriented, in-service training; individualized nature of service; and the close supervision of senior companions are also of great importance.

Where senior companions are working with terminally ill clients, the supervision is a crucial aspect. In addition to providing expertise, the supervisor must allow opportunity for the senior companions to ventilate their own feelings and must be supportive of their work. Empirical observations indicate that this supervision, if skillfully done, is not time consuming and can take place during in-service training, as well as during outgoing, regularly scheduled groups and individualized supervision.

Another key objective of the supervision of senior companions is to provide the opportunity and assistance in helping them deal with their own grief after the death of their client. Again, there is need for open discussion; opportunity for expression of grief, including crying; discussion of the invaluable contribution they made in the last days of the clients' lives; and a review of how they helped the clients and/or sometimes the bereaved families. It is most important that the project staff be available to them in what becomes a crisis in their own lives.

The program staff is able to provide these supports to the senior companions. The project is not, however, able to provide the medical supports needed. The doctors involved with the clients should be able to engage in an honest discussion with the helping persons to explain what is happening medically to the clients. Although senior companions are not expected to provide medical or nursing services, a simple understanding of what is happening to the body would be helpful. As illustrated in example 4, the senior companion herself had experienced the physical impact of chemotherapy. She was therefore able to understand what was happening to her client's body and to interpret the experience to the client and thereby reduce anxiety for both. Other senior companions do not have this personal experience and would benefit and be more effective helpers if they were given explanations. It has been suggested that simply and descriptively written pamphlets would be an aid.

On the basis of this limited experience, the authors believe that the use of oriented, skillful, and well-supervised laypersons would help alleviate the isolation experienced by dying people. A program such as the senior companion program can be effectively used in helping persons with terminal illness to remain in their own homes as long as possible. Unlike sudden death, terminal illness allows professionals, laypersons, and clients time to plan. What one does with the remaining days of a person's life assumes a unique importance under these circumstances, both to client and to senior companion.

⚔⚔⚔ 22

Dying and the Aged Person: Process and Implications for Social Work Practice

Leonie Nowitz

Very little has been written on dying and the elderly person, perhaps because everyone expects an older person to die. The assumption would thus appear to be that death is a natural and accepted process and possibly one that should be untraumatic when the dying person is an aged person.

Yet dying can be as traumatic, painful, and difficult for the older person as for anyone else. The older person has been involved in a long process in which many losses have been endured, for example, status, health, family, friends, and possibly home and financial resources. A myriad of losses usually have occurred before the final loss—of life itself—must be faced.

Recent studies, reporting a low incidence of death fear among elderly persons, support the theory that life's experiences increase the older person's capacity to cope with death. However, other factors influence a person's reaction to his own death. These include the availability of support systems or lack of them. How a person reacts to thoughts of his own death is usually similar to how he has reacted to other events in life. For an older person, the reduced resources in terms of dwindling friends and family increases his vulnerability in dealing with stressful situations. Feelings of isolation and abandonment may be intensified, particularly if the older person lives in an institution. Skilled intervention by the mental health practitioner is strongly indicated in this area. Through the presentation of my work with Mr. B., I would like to highlight some features of what dying meant to a ninety-five year-old man living in an institution and how his reactions presented problems and challenges to the practitioner involved.

Case Report

Mr. B. was born in Austria. Married at 20, he emigrated to the United States a year later. He worked as a furrier in the garment center and lived with his wife and four children. From family reports, it appears that Mr. and Mrs. B. were quite dissimilar in their interests. Mrs. B. was a warm, loving woman who was deeply religious and observed all Jewish rituals. Mr. B. was a socialist, defying religious ordinances. He was a concerned but "typically European" father, enjoying home life but involving himself in communal activities to the exclusion of his family. When his oldest daughter married, he and his wife moved into their home. While Mrs. B. was angered and embarrassed at Mr. B.'s refusing to contribute to their financial share of the household expenses, Mr. B. felt he was contributing adequately by providing babysitting services to the grandchildren.

Mr. B. left his wife and family at age 65. He went to Florida, where he remarried 13 years later. It appears that contact with his family was minimal during this period. Mr. B.'s second marriage dissolved after six years, and he blamed this on money problems. Mr. B. again left his wife but perceived both past and present instances as one in which the respective wives had left him and thus left him abandoned and "a victim of circumstances."

Mr. B. continued living in Florida despite limited income. He was planning to share an apartment with a close friend, but the friend died suddenly. Mr. B. decided to return to New York to be near his four children. His eldest daughter was unable to offer him a home, and he made his own arrangements for entering an institution. He stated that he was hoping to seek financial relief and the companionship of other people in the home.

Mr. B. was admitted to the home in 1970 and made a good adjustment. He involved himself in the home's activities and became a respected member of his community.

In the summer of 1975, Mr. B. was diagnosed as having cancer of the esophagus. He began a series of triweekly radium treatments at the nearby hospital. My services to the floor on which he lived began that December. At that time his voice was hoarse because of metastasis to his vocal cords. He became withdrawn and spent most of the time in his room. Mr. B. approached me with a laundry problem, and while we were resolving it, I began discussing his life in the home and his illness. Mr. B.'s reaction was one that was to characterize future discussions. He was angry at the doctor for not having diagnosed the tumor sooner, for he himself had suspected its presence months earlier. He blamed the doctor for taking his life away. He was also angry at two of his children, who he felt had abandoned him by relocating to Florida shortly after his admission to the home.

At the end of December Mr. B. told me that his radium treatments would be terminating shortly because the tumor had been eradicated. (The doctor later explained to me that Mr. B. had refused to continue the treatment.) He expressed several reactions:

fear of not surviving the winter because of the cold weather;

anger at the misfortune of his illness (He stated that, "If not for the tumor, I'd be a man like the others.");

projection of this anger onto the doctor for neglecting him and onto the dietitian for not providing foods that were soft and tasty; and

fear of dying expressed in his talking about the possibility of choking on his food and in his anxiety about his loss of weight.

Mr. B. told me that he had prepared his children for his death. He pointed to a list of names and phone numbers on his bureau and asked me to notify each person if he died. I agreed to do this and asked whether he really believed he would die soon. He said, "Well, maybe I'll overcome the winter." He stated that he was glad that he did not have to continue his treatments, because he would have to be exposed to the cold weather. Despite many of his fears, he remained hopeful that he would survive.

In January Mr. B. resumed his attendance at weekly floor meetings. I continued my weekly individual contacts. I discovered that his radium treatments were to be concluded in the middle of January—three weeks later than he had anticipated. When I asked Mr. B. about this, he said he was glad about the increased treatments, because he felt they were helping him. In rationalizing the treatment as beneficial Mr. B. was able to deal with his fear of debilitation and death. He continued to express his anger at the doctor, who did not pay attention to unrelated physical concerns. However, he refused my assistance in engaging the doctor to see him. He also expressed his anger at the nursing staff, whom he perceived as uncaring.

A week after termination of the radium treatments, I noticed Mr. B. was more withdrawn. He was spending increased amounts of time in his room sleeping. He explained that he was not feeling well because of the cold weather. I suggested gently the possibility of depression at the termination of treatment and fear of deterioration. Mr. B.'s response was one of anger at the staff for not being more caring, as illustrated by a wait of "several hours" to have his bed linen changed (it was only an hour); he felt he was the nurse's victim.

By reading his preadmission case material, I acquired a better understanding of his attitude. Always, it seemed, he had perceived himself as the victim of circumstances. He perceived his wife and children as leaving him, although he had left them. He told of his second wife's divorcing him, although he had left her. In approaching dying he followed a similar pattern, blaming others for the circumstances of his illness.

At the end of January Mr. B. was showing signs of physical deterioration. Bedridden with influenza, he told me one day that he was sure he would die that night. He explained that the nurse had broken his bed and that this is what would kill him. I called in the head nurse, and together we tried to understand "the broken bed." Even though neither she nor I could see where it was "broken," the nurse agreed to check out the bed with the maintenance department. Mr. B. again articulated his anger at the doctor for not visiting him. He was not specific about why he wanted the doctor but seemed satisfied that I would get him.

Increasingly depressed and withdrawn, he remained in bed and seemed to be deteriorating rapidly. His once hoarse voice became a whisper, and a new wheezing appeared in his chest, making it difficult for him to talk and to breathe. He could not speak to his daughter and son over the telephone. During a week when they could not visit him, I carried mssages between them. I began to increase my visits to several times a week and stayed for shorter periods of time as he became noticeably weaker.

On February 9 Mr. B. focused again on his anger at the doctors and nurses for not caring for him. When I acknowledged the doctor's recent presence, he said she didn't know anything. Through talking about the displeasure he had in eating, I drew out several specific problems. Mr. B. had difficulty chewing, swallowing, and digesting, and he had lost his appetite. I asked if he was worried about dying. He nodded "yes." But then he said,

"It would be better if I died. I wouldn't suffer!" (His fear of pain and debilitation may have been stronger than fear of death.) Mr. B. agreed to a psychiatric consultation to evaluate for medication to increase his appetite.

During the next week he withdrew more into sleep. When I visited, he usually woke up, and so I chose mealtimes to make my visits. Mr. B. expressed gladness that the psychiatrist had not come to see him, although the medication had not worked. I assured him it would take several weeks. We discussed specific foods that he liked and could order. I arranged for the dietitian to consult with Mr. B. to provide favorite foods. This gave him feelings of needed support and of having some control over his existence. It also demonstrated that he was being cared for.

Mr. B. continued to focus his anger on the staff and his broken bed. Later in February he told me that the head nurse was a murderess. I asked gently what had happened. He responded slowly that he had told her he was ill several weeks before, but she had ignored him. The evening nurse (whom he liked because she was warm) had called the doctor who had diagnosed that he had influenza. I responded, "So you feel *she's* killing you and not your throat." He put his hands down as if in disgust and looked away. Because of my fear that Mr. B. might distrust me or become more depressed, it was difficult for me to make the distinction concerning the "killing" agent. A few days later he woke from his sleep and whispered, pointing to his throat and then down to his chest, "It's spreading." The cancer had spread to his lungs over the last few weeks. When I asked what was spreading, Mr. B. closed his eyes and lapsed into sleep. Identifying the appropriate killing agent had given him permission to express his fears about dying of the cancer and the process it involved.

My initial reactions to Mr. B.'s deterioration were those of increased strain and sadness. The reality of his dying was becoming more obvious. He was paler, thinner, and weaker and was wheezing a great deal. It was hard for me to watch him die. I interpreted sleep as a possible withdrawal from me, rather than as a process of withdrawing from life. It was hard to witness the suffering and feel the strain in his communications with me because of the wheezing and shortness of breath. I felt helpless, angry, isolated, fearful—feelings similar to those Mr. B. had experienced. His dying was a reminder to me of my own death.

I tested the comfort of my presence with Mr. B., always asking, when he appeared to withdraw, whether he would prefer me to remain with him. I began to feel comfortable being in the room as he showed his own comfort by being able to drift into sleep and by waking up to say a few things. I began to feel closer in our relationship, in sharing his worries and his angers. At times I could not even hear the specifics of his anger, but Mr. B. seemed satisfied that I just sit and agree with him.

On February 26, Mr. B. seemed less feverish. He was sitting up, and he began talking about the doctor who had visited him that day. (Consultants were keeping a close watch.) Mr. B. stated with reassurance that the doctor said he would take care of him. He acknowledged that the doctor would not tell him what was wrong with his stomach, that is, why he could not eat. I asked if he asked the doctor what was wrong, but Mr. B. said the doctor just said he'd be OK. This indicated his feeling of being cared for and his need for hope. Mr. B. changed the topic to make specific requests for some foods. He also asked how his neighbor was, and I assured him Mr. K. was getting better. He asked me if he could get a more comfortable bed, for his was still broken. I agreed to ask the nurse about it again, and he seemed reassured. I asked if he would like fellow residents to visit. He mentioned "no," whispering that it would be too much for his voice.

Mr. B. was noticeably quieter in the first week of March. He was upset about not being oriented to time. While he thanked me for having his bed fixed (it had in fact been broken) and for collecting his spending money, he spent much of the time looking out of the window. I asked him about the faraway look on his face, and he told me that his two daughters were far away. I acknowledged that I knew from his daughter that his other daughters would be coming to see him soon. He showed no affect. Rather, he expressed concern over his bowels' not functioning well. Through exploration with the nurse it appeared that Mr. B. was focusing his anxiety about decreased food intake on decreased elimination, but he chose to see the problem as not being given adequate care by the nurse.

Mr. B.'s two daughters and son-in-law arrived from Florida on March 8. That week he showed tremendous physical improvement. He sat up in bed most of the time and directed his daughters to his concrete needs. He appeared to derive great satisfaction in his directional role, one that his daughters recollected (with humor) as a familiar personality trait in the past. Toward the end of the second week of his family's visit, Mr. B. began to withdraw. He slept more, reduced his intake of food, and at times hardly recognized his family. This was particularly stressful to his daughters as the deterioration erased any hope they might have had for his survival.

Mrs. B.'s two daughters, a son-in-law, and a granddaughter visited several times during the two weeks that they were in New York. My role was to share reactions with them about Mr. B.'s condition, work through guilt feelings of not being closer to him, help them mourn the impending loss of the father and grandfather, and concretely involve them in discussions with the medical staff to assess the metastasis.

Although both the floor doctor and the chief of the medical department acknowledged to me the seriousness of Mr. B.'s condition, both hedged on the specifics of Mr. B.'s condition when his family arrived. I later heard that the floor doctor told the family that it was Mr. B.'s depression over the daughters' abandonment of him that was causing his withdrawal from life. Thus, the doctor's inability to deal with Mr. B.'s dying caused her to deny it to Mr. B.'s family and acknowledge it only with a fellow staff member. Her inappropriate psychologizing could have had ill effects on a family that was under stress and already undergoing feelings of guilt. Fortunately, they were able to ask for my assessment of Mr. B.'s condition. While I acknowledged that I was not a medical person, I shared my personal feelings that Mr. B. was disengaging as a natural process in dying. The daughters said they had felt the same and seemed to be relieved to hear their thoughts expressed.

Because it was difficult to assess how long Mr. B. would remain in his deteriorated condition, the daughters decided to return to Florida. I accompanied them during their final visits with their father, which were extremely difficult because they did not know if they would see him again. However, neither the father nor daughters were able to acknowledge the seriousness of their farewells. Mr. B. showed little affect about his children's departure on March 23. This was due partly to his deteriorated health. His fever had increased, his weight was greatly reduced, and he could barely swallow. He said he felt as if he were in a coma, aptly describing his feeling of detachment from the world. When I asked if he was glad his children had visited, he responded slowly and almost inaudibly that he didn't care for anything except his death. The impact of the word *death* and my wish to deny it led me to hear it as—"dad, did." Mr. B. patiently corrected me. To my question, "death?" Mr. B. responded that he would be relieved to die. It would end the suffering. At this point he could not acknowledge any good or pleasurable part of his life. I shared my own feelings, that I would miss him. Mr. B. seemed to be listening. I visited Mr. B. on the morning of March 24. He pointed with great displeasure at the nursing combines that were tied around his buttocks like a diaper. He could not understand his incontinence and agreed (by nodding), while I expressed his feeling that this made him feel like a baby. He eventually calmed as I acknowledged how painful it must be for him to see his body deteriorate.

The last time I saw Mr. B. was in the afternoon of March 24. I accompanied his granddaughter into the room, and she was able to show her caring by feeding Mr. B. and telling him of her pride in his capabilities. Mr. B. expressed some caring responses to her. He died that evening in his sleep.

In assessing the impact of deterioration and impending death on Mr. B. several processes can be defined:

1. *Anger at the loss of health and independence.* Because incapacity and waning power are familiar to an older person, loss of independence and dignity may be more threatening than the concept of death (Broden, 1970).

2. *Projection of this anger* onto the milieu. This pattern of projection was an extension of Mr. B.'s coping behavior throughout his life.

3. *Fear of abandonment and isolation.* This is common among the institutionalized elderly, who have probably experienced feelings of abandonment by children at the time of choosing the institution as the last place of residence. Because of decreased physical, emotional, and concrete resources, the older person experiences feelings of vulnerability and thus feels more dependent on staff for providing caring and support. Mr. B.'s constant complaints about the lack of care from doctors and nurses spoke to his fears of abandonment and *need for support and caring.*

4. *Fear of dying.* This was demonstrated specifically by Mr. B.'s expression of his fear of choking, of losing weight, and of acknowledging that the cancer was spreading to his lungs. He also projected his fears onto the milieu in the form of the bed or of the suspicion that members of the staff were killing him.

5. *Rationalization.* Mr. B. constantly rationalized external events as being associated with his bodily functioning. Thus, if he felt ill, it was because the weather or the food was bad, not totally unrealistic elements in the etiology of his influenza or contributing factors to the difficulty in eating. This process was particularly interesting to note when the radium treatments were scheduled to stop and then were extended for a few weeks. Mr. B. rationalized each event as beneficial to him.

6. *Need for hope.* Even though Mr. B. was basically focused on his anger and was depressed, there was an occasional glimmer of hope that he might make it through the winter or that the doctors would help him.

7. *Need to be cared for.* Mr. B. constantly focused his anger on the uncaring nurses and doctors, who he reported hardly visited or showed any caring or support. Although visits were made to Mr. B., only a few

staff members were able to respond in a caring manner. The importance of medical and nursing care in restoring diminished relationships cannot be underscored enough.

8. *Depression and anxiety* about his deteriorating condition. Mr. B.'s inability to eat was felt to be more closely associated with his depression over his dying than with the cancer, according to the floor doctor. Mr. B.'s anxiety about his deteriorating health was expressed constantly. A recent study of depression in cancer patients suggests that hopelessness and loss of control are significant determinants of the ensuing depression.

9. *Organic Brain Syndrome* (OBS). Although Mr. B. was lucid most of the time, he occasionally became confused in terms of time and repeated himself. This could be attributed to a mild form of OBS.

10. *Withdrawal from the milieu.* This was noted as both a physical reaction to a deteriorating condition and a psychological need to withdraw from life. It could also be seen as a coping mechanism in the light of increased stress.

11. *Lack of need to integrate past accomplishments.* Mr. B. was too focused on his present deterioration and life situation to focus significantly on the past. His associations of the past were negative, and he stated that he could not recall or talk about past pleasures, for it took too much energy.

Whereas the social worker's own philosophy, experience, and comfort with death will help sensitize her to the experience of the client and to determine what help that client will need, the following tasks should be enumerated from my own experience.

1. I acknowledged and encouraged Mr. B.'s ventilation of anger. This took the form of projection onto the milieu for the most part, and I acknowledged past coping patterns and their obvious extension into the present situation. People handle their dying as they have handled their living. It is also possible that Mr. B.'s deterioration revived dependency feelings that stimulated anger and the safest target for discharge of these feelings was me.

2. While Mr. B. denied for the most part the source of death, he acknowledged it occasionally. I tested his reality and denial at one point when he was constantly focused on the milieu, and he expressed his fear of the spreading cancer a few days later. Although it is not necessary or even injurious at times to break a defense, I felt it might be helpful to ac-

knowledge the cancer at a strategic time to allow Mr. B. to express his fears fully. This was done in the context of a trusting relationship established between me and the client, as well as with an assessment of prior ego capacity to deal with this defense.

3. Because aged institutionalized patients *depend* on the continuity of care and familiar faces, I did several things to counteract Mr. B.'s fear of abandonment and isolation:

   A. I increased my visits and engaged myself closely in Mr. B.'s concerns, and this helped maintain a close relationship in which Mr. B. felt cared for and respected. The presence of a true ally helps to ward off confusion, maintain a dignified self-image, and encourage competent behavior and reality testing—all of which are vital objectives in attaining an acceptable death (Weisman and Kastenbaum, 1968).

   B. I reached out to staff regarding Mr. B.'s concerns, encouraging them to talk with him or asking them for things that he would like. The staff, though sympathetic, were not closely involved with Mr. B. This may be explained in part as due to their own fears of dying and their feelings of helplessness. This led them to focus on routine aspects of care rather than on developing interpersonal relationships. Mr. B. did not directly verbalize his needs to the rest of the staff and was viewed as a quiet, unresponsive patient. (Perhaps Mr. B. was afraid that direct requests for care would not be met, or perhaps he was uncomfortable at having to express his needs. He could do this through me.) Encouraging the head nurse to accompany me on specific concerns helped her experience Mr. B.'s specific difficulties. Another approach I used was to discuss Mr. B.'s difficulties and my interpretation of them with nursing and ancillary staffs to encourage interest in him. I also mentioned my own reactions to Mr. B. This met with some success with several staff members, who verbalized their reactions to Mr. B. and shared information about him.

   C. I reached for reactions in the weekly residents' group meeting about why residents were not visiting Mr. B. The discussions focused on not wanting to disturb Mr. B. A few less fearful residents did maintain contact with Mr. B., and I chatted with them from time to time about their reactions.

   D. I enlisted the help of ancillary staff—dietitian, maintenance personnel, recreation workers—to make visits and help Mr. B. with specific problems to increase his feeling of control and comfort over his milieu and give him a sense of being cared for. I also made psychiatric referrals for assessment of depression and prescription of appropriate medication.

   E. I maintained contact with the family and conveyed messages of visitation to Mr. B., which gave comfort.

4. I performed several tasks in relation to Mr. B.'s fear of dying and depression. I tried to help him maintain as much control over the process as possible by involving him in making specific requests about food, asking whether he wanted to see the psychiatrist, other residents, or his family.

5. The need to rationalize and to experience depression, anxiety, and hope are all natural reactions to the process of dying. The acknowledgment of his feelings helped him experience his reactions as ego syntonic. He felt understood.

6. One final task remained. This was the task of reviewing one's life and summing up past experiences. Despite my efforts in this direction, Mr. B. was unwilling to talk about his past. He could not make a positive use of his past accomplishments and experiences. This task is important for some older people as they face the finality of their life, but it should be started well before the final phase of dying when more energy is available to focus on the past.

In conclusion, I stress that, when an elderly person needs support during the crisis of dying, most of the staff in an institution may move away from him. This can be rationalized by the fact that society accepts an older person's death as natural and inevitable. Even when we work with elderly people facing death, we face our own feelings of vulnerability and helplessness. It is important for the social worker to be sensitive to the staff's fears and to his or her own resistances in working with a dying client.

References

Broden, A. 1970. "Reaction to Loss in the Aged." *In Loss and Grief: Psychological Management in Medical Practice,* eds. B. Schoenberg et al., pp. 199–220. New York: Columbia University Press.

Weisman, A. D. and R. Kastenbaum, 1968. *The Psychological Autopsy: A Study of the Terminal Phase of Life.* New York: Behavioral Publications.

⚞⚞⚞ Part IV
Community Resources
and Responsibilities

꧁꧁꧁ 23

Fulfillment of Life in
the Presence of Death

Irene G. Buckley

At Cancer Care, the medical component is a basis of eligibility for
our service; there must be medically determined, irreversible, advanced cancer. What is of the greatest significance (or what makes us
unique) is that our focus as a social agency is not on the *disease* itself, but on the patient and, equally, on the family, as people. In
other words, the presence of advanced cancer is just the beginning for
us; our commitment is to a view of that patient as part of a whole
social structure.

Our basic philosophy includes the enhancement of life, even in
the presence of death. Our job is to sustain the life-style of the family,
"living to the very end" for the patient and to maintain dignity,
decency, and distinction for both patient and family.

The dimensions of our responsibility consider the total social
psychological, economic, and spiritual well-being of the patient in
the site of his family at home. Many advanced cancer patients spend
a significant portion of the last days of their lives at home, where the
consequences have a potential for the most widespread damage or for
the fulfillment of life in the presence of death. Our focus is on prevention of family breakdown.

199

Cancer Care, Inc., is the service arm of the National Cancer Foundation, Inc., in the tristate New York metropolitan region. We were founded 32 years ago by a handful of volunteers who had learned through bitter experience that there was a service gap in New York City—a gap into which thousands of families fell each year. The terminal cancer patient presented a particular dilemma: there was no more medical help or medical hope. Hospitals and doctors could offer no further effective treatment. Nobody cared. However, that patient still had to be cared for until he died.

Then, as now, in the majority of cases, that patient wanted to be at home, whether he knew he was dying of cancer or not. The family wanted the patient at home in the majority of cases, too. And, in most communities, care at home, when medically sound, is frequently considered the preferred care for reasons both humane and economic.

We all realize that many families have tensions, unresolved conflicts, and difficulties in relating to each other, at best. Throw in the time bomb of advanced cancer and even the most supportive and loving of families will suffer emotionally and economically. Add to that the fact that frequently there are other illnesses existing simultaneously with cancer and you have pyramiding stresses (e.g., wife with Parkinson's disease, husband with cancer, or concurrent heart disease, diabetes, stroke, or multiple sclerosis).

A family needs help with its own totality; family members often isolate the cancer patient, making him a nonperson, owing to their guilt, denial, false hope, or a dozen other imbalances. And society walls off the family in a social quarantine mandated by fear, ignorance, superstition, and helplessness, and this occurs when patient and family are in greatest need of understanding and support!

The families who come to us are afraid, upset, and anxious. They need crisis counseling for emotional problems. Many need help on how to cope with the illness itself. Children, for example, may resent the extra attention—and money—being given to the ill member of the family or feel that somehow they are at fault for what is going wrong. Often delinquency, withdrawal, regression, or other behavioral abnormalities develop.

Our social workers provide counseling, personalized planning, and guidance tailored to each individual situation. One-to-one interviews represent the bulk of our service, but, in addition, we have organized group counseling (we have a patients' group, groups around bereavement and others). In tandem with casework planning, we also provide supplementary financial assistance in partnership with the family, for those who need it. We serve the self-supporting, middle-income group who are not eligible for government-supported services.

In 1977, we reached 25,921 people, including 7,406 advanced cancer patients. Along with the thousands of hours of the social workers' time, we helped to provide more than 760,000 hours for care at home services. The agency's total expenditures were $3,227,262, all funds coming exclusively from voluntary sources.

No age is immune to the crisis of advanced cancer. From the leukemic child to his elderly grandmother, the disease and the imminence of death take their toll. What can enrich living for a frightened, sick child or the grandmother who thinks her life should be taken instead of his? What enables the parents of this child to find joy in their other children and strength for the trial ahead?

Jimmy P. is 4½ years old, the middle child of three, friendly and active. Shortly after the birth of his 2-year-old sister, it was found that he had acute leukemia. Until recently, treatment has offered him long periods of remission during which he had a fairly normal childhood. Jimmy's parents were able to attend to the needs of all three children with time for play, love, and learning.

When the disease went out of control, Mrs. P. found herself pulled between the demands of Jimmy and her two healthy children. Even her aging mother's help with the children was not enough. Running to the hospital; coping with the anguish, the bills, the house, her family; fatigue and irritability plagued both parents and rubbed off on children with unmet needs.

The Cancer Care social worker was able to help the family select their priorities and deal with their emotions. Realizing that Jimmy and their two- and six-year-old children were more important than a clean house or perfect meals, the parents opted for a plan to protect them. The agency was able to share in the cost of a trusted babysitter who gives special attention to the children and breathing time to a worn-out mother. Mrs. P. now has the strength to devote to Jimmy and the knowledge that she is not neglecting two growing children.

Jimmy is dying but has what he needs, when he needs it most: the care of loving and restored parents, nonirritable siblings as playmates, and the unique affection of a renewed grandmother.

The future for the family should hold pride for a job well done and the rewards of two healthy children.

It is often said of the young who die: "They never had the chance to live." Perhaps there is some truth in that for the very young, like Jimmy. It is not always true of the teenager who has had the opportunity to learn, to make friends, and even to begin the process of separation from parents.

Marilyn H. was 16 years old and a junior in high school when a malignant tumor of her leg was first noted. Her parents were the victims of the Nazi holocaust; suffering and pain were no strangers to them. They had miraculously survived the concentration death camps but had lost their only son. Born just before her mother's 42nd birthday, Marilyn was pretty, bright, gifted. In short, if parents could have chosen the perfect child, they would have chosen her. She was an outstanding student with a 98.5 percent school average.

Both Marilyn and her parents refused the initial recommendation for treatment: amputation above the knee. Subsequently, she was treated with cobalt and chemotherapy. It was already apparent that Marilyn would not be a "cure."

That next summer, Marilyn was invited to a summer institute at one of the prestigious colleges and awarded a scholarship from the National Science Foundation. Ambivalent about permitting their fatally ill daughter to go away from home for the summer but wanting to do what was best for her, the parents sought help from Cancer Care, Inc.

It is easy to understand that the relationship between these parents and their only living child was unusually close. Marilyn was their "miracle" child, the child they never thought would be given to them. That she should become mortally ill—with final separation in the offing—was unbearable. They found themselves wanting to give her as normal a life as possible in the time left but not wanting to miss any precious moments with her for themselves.

The Cancer Care social worker was able to help these parents sort out their feelings, reduce their fears, and separate from their child for those precious six weeks at the summer institute. Marilyn was offered a chance to be normal while her parents experienced a trial of the ultimate separation.

Marilyn finished high school and was awarded a choice of several four-year scholarships out of town. The realistic limitation set by Marilyn and her parents was that the school chosen be no further than three hours from the treating hospital. Vassar was selected.

The parents were now able to accept this kind of separation, a gift to their daughter at a meaningful sacrifice to them.

Treatment did not halt the spread of cancer, and at the beginning of her second year in college, this lovely teenager died.

While their grief is boundless, consolation for the parents lies in the fact that they were able to provide a loving home atmosphere for their daughter and, with professional counseling, an unusually normal and productive life in the face of death.

Can anything be more devastating than to be struck with a fatal illness at the beginning of a good marriage, with young children, and with the future eagerly anticipated?

Mildred B., a 33-year-old teacher, had given up her profession temporarily to raise her children. She was happy to be at home while her husband earned the family income as an engineer. Her mother had died of breast cancer when Mildred was only 14, but Mildred retained a zest for life and hoped for a good future. Her husband, more reticent than she, was a good balance to Mildred and an anchor for this young family.

Mrs. B. had a mastectomy when her children were aged five and three. Because she needed help with the care of the three-year-old child until she could recuperate, she was referred to Cancer Care, Inc.

For a while, they managed well. They shared their concerns with the social worker and with each other and were able to deal with their children's fears about "Mommy's sickness."

When the disease spread to her spine, Mrs. B. rapidly became debilitated. She was confined to bed and could move only a few fingers. Life for them revolved around Mrs. B.'s bed. Her husband devised a special telephone through which she could talk at any time, without having to lift the receiver.

Even though paralyzed, she could continue mentally and emotionally, if not physically, to offer mothering to her children. Part-time help was no longer sufficient if Mr. B. was to continue working. Now both the children and the patient needed a great deal of physical care.

Cancer Care, Inc., secured the services of an excellent homemaker who lived in. The social worker made many home visits. Mrs. B. wanted to talk about her grief, about her physical helplessness and decline. She wanted to discuss her plans for her children and her concerns for her husband.

With the consequent relief from these anxieties, Mrs. B. was able to achieve, before she died, the deep satisfaction, that "Things would be all right."

The planning of appropriate systems for home care service is related to larger public policy issues of the day. Until we build into our health care delivery system adequate provisions for home health care, including payment for the multiple services needed at home (doctor, nurse, social worker, homemaker, and the whole array of professionals and paraprofessionals), we shall continue to give short-shrift lip service only to realizing a significant quality of life and quality health care for those coping with catastrophic illnesses.

We are not dealing with abstract theories or test tube experiments. Workers at Cancer Care have gathered monumental evidence revealing fully the benefits of organized home health care services for patients and family.

We must guarantee the inclusion of home health care service in the distribution of the national health care dollar. Such service must be available at a price we can afford. To accomplish this, we should let our voices be heard by our legislators: federal, state, and local, on behalf of our clients.

If we insist on adequate legislation and adequate insurances, we are talking about what people need, what people want, and what we know can be provided now.

≈≈≈ 24

On the Nature of Cancer:
Continuing Care of the Cancer Patient

Daniel Burdick

Currently there are more than 1.5 million Americans who have been cured of cancer, alive five years after treatment and without evidence of disease. In addition, there are 750,000 other Americans who have been treated for cancer within the last five years who will live to enter the ranks of the cured. Furthermore, with the advances in surgery, radiotherapy, hormone therapy, and chemotherapy, it is now possible to control many cancers effectively for long periods of time, during which the individual may be symptom free. Treatment for cancer may vary from the simple removal or excision of a skin cancer to the ultraradical resection for a deep-seated abdominal or pelvic tumor. Whereas surgery and radiotherapy continue to be the mainstays of cancer treatment, in recent years hormone therapy and chemotherapy have become important components of treatment. In many instances two or more treatments are used simultaneously or in sequence.

It is important to recognize three principal stages that can occur in the life history of a patient with cancer: (1) the time of primary diagnosis and institution of definitive therapy, (2) the time of possible first recurrence or metastases, and (3) the time of advanced disease.

Treatment, of necessity, varies with the stage of the disease and, more often than not, a patient receives and requires several different methods of therapy over an extended period of time during the entire course of his illness. Treatment is therefore often complex, multifaceted, and extremely costly.

With increased survival and the prolongation of life, there has developed a greater realization of the importance of how patients survive. Survival alone is not enough; the "quality of survival" has become equally important. The increasingly large number of cured or disease-controlled cancer patients constitutes a substantial rehabilitation reservoir. These patients, either because of their disease or as a result of the therapy undertaken for control of the disease, may be presented with a wide variety of problems. In addition, it must be remembered that each patient reacts to his disease in an individual manner, and his requirements for assistance and support vary accordingly. A program for rehabilitation of the patient with cancer is now considered an essential part of any hospital's or community's total cancer program. Such programs must consider the physical, functional, vocational, and sociopsychological needs of the cancer patient. Each individual who has had a mastectomy, a colostomy, a laryngectomy, or an amputation requires different kinds of assistance, instruction, and support. To deal effectively with these varied needs, a team effort is required, using medical, paramedical, and other personnel with special skills in a most efficient, cooperative manner to bring assistance and support to the cancer patient.

Unfortunately, a certain significant percent of cancer patients develop recurrence or metastatic disease at some time during their illness. When the disease becomes incurable, there is likely to be a drawn-out course in which varying periods of well-being alternate with periods of debility. The physician is called upon to institute an effective program for palliation to relieve symptoms and to slow the progressing disease. Treatments designed for palliation may be complex, and side effects can occur as a result of therapy, though these can be less severe than the symptoms they are designed to ameliorate.

No patient is beset with more anxieties, fears, and concerns than the cancer patient. Today, in most instances, the cancer patient is aware of his diagnosis. However, each patient's knowledge about cancer in general and about his illness in particular varies considerably. The cancer patient wonders whether his cancer has been eradicated and whether or not it will recur. He relates the development of any new symptom to his disease and to the possibility that this represents recurrence, until he is reassured by his physician, after adequate examination has been carried out, that no recurrence exists. If he has a physical or functional disability, he is concerned about his return to a normal productive life. If he should develop recurrence, he is concerned about the possibility of prolonged suffering or of being a burden to his family. Yet with all these anxieties, most patients exhibit remarkable courage, often in the face of incurable disease. They seem to mobilize untapped resources from within and are forever providing reciprocal encouragement to their physicians and other members of the health team.

Therefore, during the entire course of the illness, a continuum of care is required. One physician must serve as the primary, responsible person and captain of the team. The patient must sense that his doctor is fully qualified to render the treatment required and, furthermore, that he is prepared to provide continuing care throughout the illness. Intimate, meaningful relationships must be developed among the patient, the family, and all members of the medical team, to develop the feeling that support will be forthcoming whenever it is needed. A program for rehabilitation and continued care is, therefore, more than a program. It is a philosophy, an attitude of hope and encouragement that each member of the cancer team must bring to the patient—an attitude that says "This patient has a future."

In the complex, modern, stressful society in which we live, a quiet haven is necessary for effective rehabilitation. The ability of the cancer patient to adjust to his illness and to planned therapy is enhanced in the familiarity of his home environment under the skillful guidance and compassion of his medical team and family.

ᏔᏔᏔ 25

Homemaker-Home Health Aides— Essential Thanatologists

Florence M. Moore

The K.'s are in their 80s. She has breast cancer, inoperable because of her age, and a cardiac condition. He has stomach cancer and is on chemotherapy. A full-time homemaker has been able to care for them and nursing home placements were averted (Statement by National Cancer Foundation and Cancer Care, Inc., 1975).

These four sentences sketch a poignant family situation in which homemaker-home health aide service contributed to the care at home of two terminally ill persons. There are thousands of situations involving individuals of all ages where homemaker-home health aide and other in-home services can help prevent or delay final institutional care and can also provide valuable help following death.

One cannot overstate the importance of having a calm, security-giving, caring figure in the home when a family member has a terminal illness. This is especially important where there are children and the terminally ill person is the mother. A homemaker-home health aide, the paraprofessional member of the helping team, can hold a family together in the security of their familiar home surroundings. Taking on such everyday duties as preparing meals, making beds, shopping, doing the dishes and laundry, being there when the children get home from school, and supervising their homework can help to cushion the terrifying impact of terminal illness. Emotional support is another key function of this individual. In fact, the presence of a mature, supportive homemaker-home health aide can assist both the father and the children by sharing their burden of grief. Children especially need someone who can listen to their fears while still helping them go on with the business of living. The loss of a parental figure, particularly a mother, can scar children for life. Preventive help given them at this crucial and traumatic period can prevent serious emotional problems from developing then or later on.

The orderly operation of a household can itself help to create a peaceful environment and be very comforting and supportive to a husband and father overburdened with worry about his wife's illness and medical bills. Without adequate help adults, as well as children, can break down under the terrible strain of the terminal illness of a loved one.

Of enormous social significance is the fact that families who are separated during crises frequently never get back together—or take months or years to do so. The presence of the homemaker-home health aide to act as a mother substitute during this grievous period may prevent the further trauma of loss of contact among other family members.

One of the great strengths of the use of these paraprofessionals is that, like a mother, they can assist with personal care, as well as with care of the household. For example, with proper training and supervision, they can assist the patient with a bath, care for hair and teeth, help with toileting, care for the bed and bedroom, and undertake other tasks that save valuable time of more costly and frequently scarce professional personnel, and they can be taught to observe changes in the patient's condition or in the family relationships and report these to the professional members of the team who are responsible for the plan of care.

It has been shown at least in one study (American Cancer Society, 1974) that, next to family members, it is the homemaker-home health aide with whom the patient may feel most comfortable about discussing concerns crucial to himself and his family. In such situations the paraprofessional staff member is the bridge between the patient and the professional members of the team.

When the terminally ill patient is a child, a homemaker-home health aide may be needed to help the mother with her usual household duties and the care of other children so that she may spend some time with the ill child. Or the homemaker may be needed to assist the mother with the care of the ill child so that she can give essential attention to other children in the family. In still other cases, the mother of a terminally ill child may need a period of respite for the protection of her own physical and emotional health.

For all members of the health team strong support must be available at all times. This is particularly important for the homemakers, however, who do not have professional knowledge to fall back on. They need not only this support but also immediate access to it and to guidance as well. Furthermore, the agency employing the homemaker-home health aide should give very careful consideration to the advisability of assigning an individual, without respite, to one case after another involving great emotional stress. Careful thought must be given to what continual emotional strain and drain may do to the emotional and physical health of the aide herself. It may be essential for certain individuals to have assignments such as these spaced out.

It is always important that the paraprofessional be recognized as a full member of the health and social service team. This is particularly true when it involves patients who are terminally ill because it establishes, in a very concrete way, that the problems of the patients and family are not borne solely on the shoulders of the paraprofessional. Rather, they are shared with other responsible, caring persons.

The need for quality service in such trying circumstances as terminal illness should be abundantly clear. The National Council for Homemaker-Home Health Aide Services has developed standards and has in operation a voluntary national service-monitoring system. Fourteen basic standards have been established and 92 programs have been found to be in substantial conformity with these standards.

Basic National Standards for Homemaker-Home Health Aide Services

1. The agency shall have legal authorization to operate.
2. There shall be an appropriate duly constituted authority in which ultimate responsibility and accountability are lodged.
3. There shall be no discriminatory practices based on race, color, or national origin, and the agency either must have or be working toward an integrated board, advisory committee, homemaker-home health aide services staff, and clientele.
4. There shall be designated responsibility for the planning and provision of financial support to at least maintain the current level of service on a continuing basis.
5. The service shall have written personnel policies; a wage scale shall be established for each job category.
6. There shall be a written job description for each job category for all staff and volunteer positions which are part of the service.
7. Every individual and/or family served shall be provided with these two essential components of the service:
   A. Service of a homemaker-home health aide and supervisor
   B. Service of a professional person responsible for assessment and implementation of a plan of care.
8. There shall be an appropriate process utilized in the selection of homemaker-home health aides.
9. There shall be: (A) initial generic training for homemaker-home health aides such as outlined in the National Council For Homemaker Services' training manual; (B) an ongoing in-service training program for homemaker-home health aides.
10. There shall be a written statement of eligibility criteria for the service.
11. The service, as an integral part of the community's health and welfare delivery system, shall work toward assuming an active role in an ongoing assessment of community needs and in planning to meet these needs, including making appropriate adaptations in the service.
12. There shall be an ongoing agency program of interpreting the service to the public, both lay and professional.
13. The governing authority shall evaluate through regular systematic review all aspects of its organization and activities in relation to the service's purpose(s) and to the community needs.
14. Reports shall be made to the community, and to the national council for homemaker-home health aide services, as requested.

Key items in these standards include careful selection of the homemaker-home health aide, provision of initial generic training before she goes on duty, regular ongoing in-service training sessions and supervision by appropriate professionals. The other National Council standards have to do with personnel practices, job descriptions, budgets, community planning, reporting, civil rights, and others. The National Council submits that all of these standards, but particularly those on training and supervision, must be met if homemaker-home health aide service is to provide therapeutic caring service that will assist a terminally ill person so that he can die with dignity at home.

The National Council believes that, to ensure quality care, every homemaker-home health aide program should have its standards of service checked on a regular, continuing basis through an objective review. This principle is *not* adhered to routinely at this time in the homemaker-home health aide service field. There are many agencies, including a growing number of proprietary agencies, delivering this vitally needed service that, in effect, are responsible to no one but themselves. Appropriate actions by knowledgeable individuals can help to shape the climate for ensuring high-quality in-home service for terminally ill persons and for their families, as well as for others.

These would include actions based on principles such as:

1. National basic standards should be agreed upon for the field.
2. Each service, regardless of auspice, should be accountable to the public by undergoing, on a regular basis, an objective review of its standards of operation.
3. Homemaker-home health aides should receive initial generic training and continuing in-service training.
4. Homemaker-home health aides should be an integral part of the health and social service team and should be supervised by appropriate professional persons.

A significant factor of great concern to the individuals and families involved in what may be a long-term illness are the costs of care. Ruth Howard, a 36-year-old Massachusetts mother of two, has a deep-seated, inoperable, and growing brain tumor. She has become an ardent crusader for a national health insurance plan that would protect middle-income families like her own against breakup caused by catastrophic illness. She has even testified before the House Ways and Means health subcommittee. This courageous young woman has said of her own situation:

People opposing legislation to lower the cost of homemaker services say that someone in the family can always take care of the kids. And so who do you get to help? Both sets of grandparents in our family are very energetic and very terrific, but after a week and a half of running this household, it was all over. They just had to get out of here. The fact is, you need someone who is trained to take care of the situation where there is a lot of panic and upset. The kids are the most important part of this and if it happens that I am in bed for a good year before I die, we're going to need a homemaker and have this backup of holding and loving and calmness and taking care of things.

Usually, home care and homemaker-home health aide service is less costly than institutional care, but, even so, long-term or intensive need for service can put a severe financial drain even on middle-income families.

In-home service maximizes what the family and patient can do for themselves, but currently, the health system is institution oriented. The funding mechanisms are primarily geared to hospital and nursing home care. The scope of coverage for in-home services is very limited. At times the services that the patient needs, including "homemaker" services, are not included as covered benefits. This is true not only of major government programs such as Medicare and Medicaid but also of the insurance industry, which models its programs after Medicare. A national policy supportive of home care is the only answer. The in-home aspect of the service continuum must be fully recognized in any national health insurance plan.

Homemaker-home health aide service is a vital member of the family of in-home services. Homemaker-home health aides are essential thanatologists. Homemaker-home health aide service is needed in its own right for many dying patients. It can also facilitate the delivery, in the home, of professional services. This discussion of its usefulness is based on the premise that the service to be given will be a high-quality service. All those involved in thanatology can be of great assistance in seeing that this vital in-home service is available in each community so that it will be there to help in the tremendously sensitive and emotion-laden time of terminal illness.

References

American Cancer Society, New York State Division, Rochester, New York. 1974. Summary of "Home Care of the Cancer Patient. I. Report of Pilot Study on Patient and Family Opinion." October.

National Cancer Foundation and Cancer Care, Inc. 1975. Statement on Certain Medicare Issues to Representative Dan Rostenkowsky, Chairman, Subcommittee on Health, House Ways and Means Committee, September 19.

⩗⩗⩗ 26

The Community Center in the Life of a Dying Person with No Family Involvement

Herbert Hildebrandt

For the dying person to remain at home, a support system offering that particular choice is needed. Traditionally, this kind of system has been found within the patient's own family. However, the mobility of our society often means that the family is scattered or, in many cases, people have never married or have outlived their children. Institutionalization appears to be the only alternative open to the person who lives alone.

At the Stanley M. Isaacs Neighborhood Center (New York City) we are attempting to provide an alternative to enable the dying person to remain at home. The care system, located at the center, involves seven different services that work with older people. The system works with the ambulatory as well as the homebound, and it recognizes that there is a progression from one to another. This community center includes the following services:

1. A senior citizens' day center, used by between 250 and 300 people daily, is operated by the Department of Social Services.

2. An outreach clinic of New York Hospital, staffed by doctors, nurse practitioner, nurses, and a social worker five days a week at the Center, provides medical evaluation and continuing treatment.
3. An outreach program, called Search and Care, deals with the homebound people of the area, providing such services as counseling, housekeeping, shopping, escort, and dealing with the other agencies involved in the person's life.
4. A meals on wheels program delivers 200 meals daily to homebound people in the area. This program also employs a social worker who deals with such problems as housekeeping, shopping, and escort.
5. Two resident social workers, living in the housing project where the center is located, are available 24 hours a day 7 days a week. They also provide services to the older population similar to those already noted.
6. A telephone reassurance program calls homebound people each day to check on their condition and also to provide additional services when needed.
7. A hospital provides doctors for psychological evaluation and consultation, when requested.

These seven services have been organized in a small area of the Upper East Side of Manhattan. As we organized them, we often found that several services were working with the same clients, and there was often duplication of services. To avoid this and also to achieve greater clarity in the assessment of the client situation, we began to merge the seven services into one single system of care. Working with New York Medical College, we began to design a central status form to be used by all services. The form reflects the client's history, current situation, areas in which work is being done, and those problems which have been solved and the method of solution.

All services meet once a week for client review, as well as for educational meetings with outside speakers. The form also designates a primary case manager. This is a worker from one of the seven services who assumes overall responsibility for the case. Other services involved with the client always refer to the primary case manager and give feedback on their contacts with the client.

The status form lists ten target areas in which work for the client is carried on, as follows: (1) physical; (2) emotional; (3) activities of daily living such as shopping, escort, and bill paying; (4) family; (5)

leisure and associates; (6) housing; (7) finance; (8) vocational and educational; (9) legal; and (10) other general.

The target codes include "Declare and intention to do something—Find out, Entailed," in which a problem exists but a remedy is lacking (such as the client's having a physical disability); and "Get on with it," in which a worker is telling himself to move on a previously declared intention.

Dispositions reflect those problems which have been solved and the resources used to solve them. A status form is entered on each client of the seven services, and a central file is established that is available to all workers within the care system. A new worker reading the file will see where the client has come from, where he is now, what problems exist, and what problems have been solved. Through New York Medical College we have been able to computerize these forms, and we are now beginning to receive aggregate data on our population. We have received demographic data, an analysis of target, and disposition areas.

The demographic data indicate 68 percent of our population live alone, 46 percent are widowed, 14 percent were never married, and 8 percent are divorced or separated. In addition, some 77 percent of the population is female, 10 percent are between 55 and 64 years of age, 32 percent between 65 and 74, 31 percent between 75 and 84, and 8 percent between 85 and 94 years of age.

An analysis of the areas targeted for our intervention shows the following ranking order: (1) activities of daily living, (2) physical, (3) emotional, (4) leisure time fillers, (5) finance, (6) housing, (7) familial, (8) legal, (9) vocational and educational.

In terms of dispositions, we have been most successful in the area of activities of daily living, which include such things as shopping, escort, and housekeeping. We have "entailed" physical to the same degree in which we have "declared intentions." This indicates a large number of chronic physical problems that have been treated medically but for which no further medical treatment is possible. It has been estimated that between 60 and 70 percent of the people 65 years of age and older suffer from some form of chronic illness. As their illness progresses, their world constricts and their dependency on others increases.

The following case history reflects how the system of care has enabled an individual to remain in his own home. Harry lived in the housing project in which the center was located. He has never married and has been on disability for approximately 10 years. The first status form submitted indicated that he was a "loner" and that this was important to him. He had a brother, but he chose not to have any contact with him. He had one or two friends whom he would meet but who never came to his apartment. He came to the center each day for lunch. He would stand outside until it was served, go in and eat, then leave immediately when he had finished. He said that he could not stand the crowd for any length of time. I would see him each day standing outside the center and would stop for a brief chat. One day he indicated to me that he was dissatisfied with the medical care that he was receiving at a local hospital, and I suggested that he try the clinic at the center. I took him in and introduced him, and they took over his care. At this point he was involved with the community center to a limited degree, for example, telephone reassurance and the clinic. Because the clinic was the most active at this time, its staff became primary case managers.

The next status form indicated that the clinic had determined that his condition was indeed chronic and progressive. He was given medication to help ease the pain during attacks, a supply of oxygen, and assistance in obtaining an air conditioner to help him through the summer. When he complained about the noise in the building, which disturbed him during his attacks, he was helped to file an application for a senior citizen house, but he was told that his chances for getting in were limited.

The next status form expressed his concern over the loss of his friend, whom, as his attacks increased in frequency and severity, he was unable to get out to meet. The friend would not come to his home, and Harry's isolation became greater. I spoke to the friend and asked him to visit. He did once, but I felt that when he looked at Harry, he saw himself and could not take it. I had other people visit and increased the number of telephone calls, but these efforts did not really help him much. I spoke to him about a nursing home where the chances of socialization were more positive, but he refused even to think about this.

The next status form showed that his condition was deteriorating and that the clinic had done as much as it could for him. It was decided to place him on "meals on wheels," and telephone reassurance was designated as the primary case manager. It was arranged with meals on wheels that, if he could make it down to the center for lunch, they would hold his meal. With time he came down to the center less and less frequently. In a talk with the clinic social worker he said he knew he was dying but that he thought dying would not be so hard.

The work then became one of maintenance. We would call him in the morning, and the meal would be delivered at noon. He became less interested in having visitors, but I would go up occasionally and talk for 15 minutes, which was all that he could take. Once a week a teenager would do whatever shopping had to be done. Whatever cleaning he wanted done he managed to do himself. He always wore pajamas now.

One day he did not answer our morning call. I called the police, and we broke in. He was lying by the door as if he were trying to get out. The ambulance crew came, revived him, and rushed him to the hospital. The doctors said that he should be placed in a home, but he died the following day.

Harry had been known to the care system for a number of years, and just as importantly he knew the system. He had come to the center each day; for three years we called him each morning; for two years the clinic tried to ease his dying; for one year meals on wheels helped to feed him. Harry knew us, and we knew him. He would talk to us, and we would listen, and he would listen to us.

As his needs increased, the resources to meet them were found within the care system that he knew and had confidence in. Because the workers were part of a system, they talked to each other, a consistent approach was established, and new needs were easily communicated. Harry chose to die without his family, and it was the comprehensive community-based care system that helped him to remain in his own home until the end.

The care system itself could meet Harry's needs. However, this is often not the case, and outside agencies must be sought for additional help, such as housekeepers, homemakers, and home attendants. These workers are provided by agencies outside the system, and coordination is often difficult. The dying person may display anger or be difficult to please, resulting in constant staff changes. If the worker could be integrated into our care system, greater understanding could be provided for both the worker and the client. The center is presently attempting to establish a program in which we will hire, orient, train, and place the housekeepers with the dying client. The staff person will introduce the worker to the client and will be available to resolve disputes as they arise.

Although many of our clients use the clinic at the center, there are many who use other medical facilities in the area. The dying person often spends a good deal of time in a hospital. The workers within the care system have tried to coordinate their efforts with the medical facility; however, this often does not work. We make the hospital staff aware of our involvement so that we can be included in discharge planning, but this too does not always work. A hospital recently sent a patient who had suffered a massive stroke home to a fifth-floor walkup and left her there. Although we try to keep a check on our people, it was a day before the care system was reinstituted. We are trying to create a closer working relationship with the other institutions in our area, but it is often a difficult job.

The New York Medical College has opened a Center for Comprehensive Preventive Care. This will offer a team approach to providing primary medical care. The team will include doctors, psychologists, psychiatrists, social workers, and other specialists. Especially important for the dying patient is the plan for all of these people to make home visits. We will, for the referrals that we make to this center, become part of the team; we will be involved in all aspects of case planning.

The person who is dying at home is often restricted to that home. All services must be brought to him, and they must somehow fill the 24 hours in a day. I recently did a survey among the homebound people with whom we work, and I found that on average they slept some four hours per night. They would go to bed at 10 P.M. and wake up at 2 A.M.; they would go to the bathroom and then return to bed. All of them turned out the lights, and they would lie there and the night would magnify their condition and amplify the sounds that threatened them. Each person on the telephone reassurance was asked what time of day they wished to be called, and all responded "in the morning" as a confirmation that they had made it through the night.

The dying person quickly establishes a routine of living. Each day is the same: get up, wash, eat, watch TV, clean, and sleep. The routine in itself is debilitating. The center plans to obtain a vehicle that can be used to break the isolation of the dying person by taking him to the park or letting him pick out his own chicken for supper.

In several cases the dying person did have family members, but they were unable to deal with the approaching death. Through the dying person the family came to know us and to see us as a resource to deal with the business aspects of dying. This includes making of wills and dealing with the other agencies involved in the dying person's life. Often the family came to us to try and gain some understanding of what was happening to their dying family member. Often the approaching death creates conflict within the family. The families have exhibited feelings of anger, guilt, rejection, and inadequacy over the impending death. Through the center's agreement with a family counseling agency, our referrals have been accepted, and help is given to families to deal with these problems.

We have a senior companion program in which older people visit, on a regular basis, the homebound people in the area. In those cases where the client was dying the family often used the senior companion to try to gain a further understanding of what the older person was going through.

The staff members of the care system would take over the business aspects of dying, and this would enable the family members to cope with the emotional problems. They could learn not to relate differently to the family member now that he was dying and to gain greater confidence in being with the dying person. The care system would never try to replace the family; rather, it tried to help both the family and the dying person to deal with the death.

In summary, the role of the community center care system in the life of the dying person is to ease the living of the dying person. The system is aware of his needs and is aware as these needs increase. Clients have often said that someone was up to see them, but they did not know who they were, what they wanted, or where they came from. The care system is trying to eliminate this uncertainty by providing greater coordination of services. It is also trying to expand the programs to offer the services to more people. On one occasion an elderly woman was found who had been dead for two weeks. A center member said to me that it was really a shame that nobody had missed her during all that time.

It is the role of the primary case manager to coordinate the care given within the system and also to relate to the providers from outside agencies. In part, it is an attempt to see a living person with a past, present, and future—not a dying person. Often providers see a fractionated person: the doctor sees a medical problem; the social worker, a social security problem; and the housekeeper, a urine-soaked sheet. It is the system's function to get them to see a whole person and to judge the needs in this context. The center is attempting to increase the services that it directly provides with the goal of creating greater rationality of care.

This center has been in existence for 10 years. We have provided for clients' recreational needs, and when illness comes, other parts of the care system become involved. Many of the active members have said that, above all, they never want to be sent to a nursing home. We have respected this wish and have fought to keep them in their own home. We are attempting to create a total care system that recognizes who the person was, who he is now, and what his particular needs are. In those cases where there is a family we assume a secondary role; when the person is alone, we assume greater responsibility. Often, we can do little to prevent a death, but at least we can try to add some comfort to the life of the dying person.

27

Comprehensive Planning for Care and the Home Health Agency

Isabelle M. Clifford

Comprehensive planning for care of the terminal patient and his family should start at the time of diagnosis and continue through all stages of the illness. It includes planning for hospitalization and for out-of-hospital care. Much concern has been evident in recent years over the right of a terminal patient and/or his family to choose how and where he is to spend the months or days remaining to him. Should he be in a facility specializing in care that meets his medical needs but restricts his personal life? Or should his desire to be at home with his family be facilitated by the availability of appropriate in-home care? If he chooses the latter, how comprehensive is the planning for home health care?

There are many facets to a comprehensive planning process that begin before such a decision is made. All too frequently the focus has been on the patient's continuing medical care. The need for this is not questioned, but the process should include other vital aspects, such as:

1. counseling the patient and his family members, not only about medical care, but also about social and psychological needs and planning for the future;

2. preparation of personnel involved with the patient for the emotional and psychological impact of caring for him;
3. preparation of the patient and family for the transition from institutional to home care;
4. communication, predischarge and continuing, with the primary source of home health care;
5. planning by home care personnel with the patient and family for home health care.

If quality of life is a prime consideration, all these factors must be included in a comprehensive coordinated plan of care that is geared to individual needs. It is essential that all concerned have input into such a plan—the attending physician, consultants, hospital services, and home health personnel. Of special importance is the inclusion of the patient and the family in the planning process. A cooperative effort in the planning stage leads to better understanding and implementation of the plan. It also leads directly to the enhancement of the quality of life for the terminal patient and to needed support for the family.

The patient with a terminal illness and his family have many concerns, especially during hospitalization, when diagnosis and prognosis are determined. Among them are: (1) the immediate present and how to cope with their feelings, (2) the time remaining to the patient and what will happen to him, (3) the ability of the family to manage, (4) the approaching death and what it will mean to the family. Comprehensive planning includes attention to these concerns as they arise during this crucial period for the patient and his family.

Counseling is imperative if the quality of life is to be enhanced and maintained at an optimal level. It should begin at the time of diagnosis and should continue through all stages of illness. Counseling should be directed toward the concerns mentioned and should be extended to preparation for death and its aftermath. The patient needs to feel that he is in control and able to direct the disposal of his estate whether of financial or sentimental value. He may also have some definite ideas regarding the type of funeral and possibly the donation of body parts for humanitarian reasons. He may have already made some arrangements that should be discussed with family members. A counselor, particularly a clergyman, may be of special value in facilitating such discussion. Other counseling services may be available, people who are trained to give professional help, who can identify problem areas, draw out hidden concerns, and skillfully initiate helpful discussion.

In the process of planning, it must be recognized that many individuals have an influence on the environment of the patient. These range from the nursing staff and volunteers to the cleaning woman and the television man in the hospital and include all personnel who come in contact with the patient and family at home. All of these individuals should be guided in providing a 24-hour milieu of support and reassurance. Little does the healthy individual appreciate the demoralizing effect on the patient of a thoughtless remark made directly or loud enough to be overheard, or of body language that clearly speaks of rejection to the patient. Appropriately trained, however, these individuals can exert a very effective and positive influence through tone of voice and thoughtful little gestures and actions. Reassurance is important for all patients, but it is of special value to those terminally ill. Explaining procedures beforehand and letting him know what to expect are most helpful. Of special value is giving the patient opportunities to express his anxieties. All too frequently he feels cut off and isolated with a sense of not being involved in his own care.

Preparation of personnel involved with the patient does not end with factors influencing a good environment for the patient. It must be directed toward the individual attitude toward death. Can each individual accept death as an ultimate for himself? Can each be comfortable in caring for or coming in contact with a terminal patient? If not, the quality of life for that patient during his remaining time will be diminished. Help must therefore be provided in facing the fact that death is a part of living. Opportunities for discussing this issue and for guidance in resolving it are necessary in comprehensive planning for care of the terminally ill.

Trauma to varying degrees caused by relocation has been experienced by everyone. This may have been a geographic relocation to an entirely new situation with different living and working patterns and separation from the security of family and friends. It may have been a move to another neighborhood involving a search for new shopping, banking, and service sources. Each change has had its effect.

Think of the trauma of relocation to the terminal patient! He is usually admitted hastily to the hospital, perhaps for the first time in his life, with no preparation for an alien setting. Although little can be done about admission, much can be done during hospitalization through counseling and reassurance. The patient and his family get to know hospital personnel and to feel secure within the institutional setting. Then they become concerned with cost of institutional care and with limited privacy and develop mixed feelings around returning home. It is important to recognize the need for preparing both the patient and the family for the patient's return home in such a manner as to reassure them of continuity of care and to minimize the trauma of relocation.

The patient may be reluctant to leave the security of the hospital, where trained people known to him are readily accessible to meet his needs. He may be unfamiliar with the services of a home health care program and the qualifications of its personnel. Although he wants to go home, he may not trust his family's ability to cope with his illness. He may also be greatly concerned with the acceptance of others if he had undergone surgery that has changed body functioning or caused visible disfigurement.

The family, although wishing for opportunities to express affection or to make plans in privacy, has its own concerns regarding their ability to cope with patient care and change in living pattern. They, too, may have questions regarding home health personnel's ability to meet their needs, such as instruction, counseling, and reassurance. They may also have doubts about facing up to disfigurement and changed body functioning.

If a beginning is not made in the hospital to cope with the trauma of relocation with both the patient and his family, severe problems will develop in the home. They should be prepared for the kinds of help that will be available to them there. They should know who is coming and why. The family needs to be involved in the planning process, and the patient should be brought in as much as possible. It is also vital that home health personnel recognize their responsibility to continue coping with the trauma of relocation.

Of great help in minimizing the stress of returning home is making arrangements to meet individual needs before actual discharge. This includes use of all community resources that can be effective in ensuring appropriate care. A multidiscipline team effort is required, preferably with a home health service program functioning as the primary source of home care. When special techniques are involved, the home care personnel can come to the hospital for demonstration and instruction. This will ensure better continuity and quality of care. When necessary, an assessment of the home situation may be indicated. From this a better picture is gained about the ability of the family to care for the patient, the accessibility of a responsible person, and the housing and environmental conditions. All of these may be determining factors in the decision whether home care is appropriate or not. Ideally, this home assessment should be made for all patients before discharge. Practically, it is impossible.

A bridge of communication between hospital and the home health agency must be established with two-way communication between personnel of both agencies. This is of particular importance in the planning stage for transition from hospital to home. The home health agency knows community services available. Joint planning facilitates better care at home and enhances opportunities to improve the quality of life for the patient and his family.

Other arrangements for services not provided through the local home health program should be made before discharge. These include arranging for all types of appropriate in-home support services, such as homemaking, transportation, meals, barber or beautician, personal contacts, and pastoral services.

A most vital aspect of arrangements for followup care is that of having all needed equipment in the home before the patient arrives there. Equipment, such as a hospital bed, bedpan, raised toilet seat, tub and toilet rails, and commode, may be essential for the family in caring for the patient. Specialized treatment equipment for stoma care, catheter irrigation, and so forth, must be in the home if continuity of care is to be sustained. An ample supply of dressings, ointment, and/or medications should be provided as appropriate. Lack of any essential item is most distressing to family members already unsure of their ability to meet the patient's needs, and it adds to the patient's feeling of insecurity. These items are also necessary if the home health personnel are to proceed effectively with prescribed treatment.

The home health agency has other important needs if it is to provide continuity and quality of care. Information transmitted from the hospital must be comprehensive, giving all data pertinent to total patient care. There are rarely difficulties with diagnosis, vital statistics, and kind of treatment to be given. However, it is frequently unclear who is to give the treatment in borderline areas of service functioning, such as in ambulation exercises and activities of daily living—the nurse or the physical therapist. The referral should clearly spell out when such activities require the special skills of the physical therapist. This information may aid the home care program in obtaining the personnel required to fill demands for service.

It is essential that the home health nurse know all medications that the patient is taking, whether oral or given by injection. If by injection, the frequency, dose, and site must be clearly noted. Information regarding potential side effects and the procedures to counteract these is vital, not only to ensure quality of care, but also to enable the nurse to reassure the patient and family when drug reactions do occur.

All home health personnel need to know what the patient has been told of his condition and his reaction and what has been told to the family. This is necessary for continuing reassurance and counseling. It also helps in avoiding any damaging "slips" of information because of a lack in communication. It is imperative that home health personnel know what the patient and family members have been taught regarding treatment procedures. One cannot assume that certain teaching has been done in the hospital because it is accepted standard practice. Circumstances may have prevented this, or it may have been incomplete. There may have been incomplete or poor understanding by the patient and family that restricts their ability to put this knowledge into practice at home. If the home health staff is to provide continuity, they must be able to pick up where the hospital left off, perhaps even retrace some steps for better understanding. This not only enhances the effectiveness of care but also is a prime factor in establishing rapport with the patient and family.

Discharge planning must include the establishment of a two-way communication system. One person in the hospital and one in the home health agency should be designated as coordinators who accept the responsibility for clarifying treatment orders, sharing information, solving problems, and keeping both agencies aware of the current situation. This is imperative if the hospital is providing specialized treatments.

The home health agency has a responsibility to report back to the referring agency results of home visits, problems that should be brought to the physician's attention, status of the patient, and the family situation. Since continuing assessments are made of patient needs in his home situation and of the family strengths and weaknesses, additional services may be recommended. These may be services that were not anticipated at time of discharge but that will contribute to better total patient care. They may also be necessary to minimize additional stress on other family members. Without a system of communication and coordination, it might be difficult to implement these recommendations. Quality of life for both patient and family could then be at less than a desirable level.

The home health agency should coordinate its calls, whether to the physician or to the designated coordinator. Consideration must be given to the amount of time involved in responding to requests so that the burden does not destroy the effectiveness of the communication system.

Home health personnel have many questions that need answers so that a total home care plan may be developed. These answers must be available before the patient and family are brought into the planning process and before the first home visit is made. Of prime importance in all cases are the awareness of the patient and the family's attitudes toward the terminal illness, their level of acceptance. Are they able to discuss this among themselves, with others? Or are they aware of the outcome and refuse to discuss it? The home care staff can then be guided in an appropriate approach with them.

If there has been a mastectomy, have breast forms been discussed, perhaps demonstrated, and has information been given on adaptations possible, as well as on commercial sources? The quality of life can be greatly enhanced if a woman can feel she looks feminine. Has she been given instruction on adaptation of clothing? She should be encouraged to maintain as near normal activity as long as possible. This includes going to church and to visit family. She needs to feel that she is well dressed despite her "disfigurement." Is edema present? What measures were taken in the hospital to reduce it? Was the individual measured for a pressure sleeve? What instructions were given about putting the sleeve on correctly? When and how long should she wear it? How much nerve damage, if any, occurred? Does the physician recommend physical therapy to improve or maintain shoulder-arm function? How is her husband accepting the situation? Is social service needed? Has there been metastasis to the long bones? If so, safety precautions need to be exercised to prevent fractures, which are another blow to patient/family stability. Knowledge of bone structure is essential, even when the patient is just getting out of bed.

What teaching has been done with the individual with a laryngectomy or a tracheostomy? Was a humidifier recommended to help avoid crusting? Is nutrition counseling needed to consider what foods are acceptable and palatable? A blender may be recommended for foods when there are problems with swallowing and with jaw and tongue action, but what if there is no electricity in the home? The nutrition consultant can suggest other means of accomplishing the same purpose—specific kinds for specific needs. Other information helpful to the nutritionist include details about surgery, about whether or not any tastebuds are left, and about the effect on olfactory nerves that affect appetite. Are there other problems such as cardiac involvement or diabetes? Is the cardiac patient taking a diuretic? If so, which one, so that food and drug interactions can be avoided and electrolyte imbalance prevented?

Home health personnel—the nurse, the physical therapist, the nutritionist, the social worker, and others—are all concerned with the emotional aspect. They realize how greatly the illness affects the home situation and vice versa perhaps better than institutional personnel. They recognize the problems of body image. With as much background information as possible made known to them, they can be much more supportive.

With a comprehensive referral the home care staff and the patient and his family together can develop a plan for home care and can work toward its implementation. This joint process helps build a meaningful and trusting relationship. The patient and his family need to feel they have some control over what occurs in their own home. Yet they appreciate the guidance and support in maintaining the needed level of care. It is essential that the home health personnel schedule their visits as much as possible to meet the needs of the situation. Time should be allowed for the patient and family members to vent their anxieties.

In conclusion, quality of care and quality of life can best be achieved through (1) comprehensive planning for all stages of illness, (2) counseling and preparation of both patient/family and of personnel having contact with them, (3) a good communication system for the provider of care, and (4) coordination of all aspects of care; institutional, community, and home. Above all, the focus of attention must be on the individual and family needs.

≈≈≈ 28

Shall We Look Before We Leap?

Stanley Budner

Home care for the dying patient represents, in good part, home care for the cancer patient. Cancer is often viewed as a sentence of death, and for approximately two out of three cancer patients, this is the reality. The length of time between diagnosis and death for these patients is variable, but for many it is relatively long, more than six months. The degree to which this time is spent in hospitals is also variable, depending on the nature and course of the disease, the physician, the patient, and family, but for many it is only a relatively small proportion of the total time involved. Thus, even though care of the cancer patient is often seen as inseparable from hospitalization, home care already constitutes a large part of the reality of treatment for incurable cancer patients.

However, it is one thing to accept the fact that home care for the cancer patient is a de facto component of cancer care, another to establish it as an explicit, formal program. Even though the quality of patient care in our hospitals, especially the care provided the dying patient, leaves much to be desired, there are risks in a simple comparison between the deficiencies of a system actually in operation and the best we hope to achieve with a system yet to be tried or even developed. Since change has its costs and reforms do not always work out as anticipated, perhaps we should look at what we may actually accomplish, as well as at what we hope to achieve before we leap. Such a look might persuade us to change our minds about the desirability of developing new approaches and should certainly help us maximize the benefits obtained and minimize the costs involved.

Of course, I ignore my own admonition, to look before you leap, by jumping to the benefits of home care before looking at the pitfalls.

The Leap

There appear to be many reasons why home care for the incurable cancer patient should be considered desirable. Because modern hospitals are designed to provide very specialized environments for treating those health problems which require sophisticated personnel and technology, hospitalization is of necessity a costly option, one that can be justified only when the specialized resources of hospitals must be brought into play. If a patient is kept in the hospital after the need for these specialized resources is past or is hospitalized for other reasons, then an economic burden is imposed on the patient and his family and a social waste is created through the irrational allocation of scarce resources.

In addition, from the viewpoint of the patient, hospitalization entails a disruption of the normal pattern of relationships with and support by the family, as well as a separation from the security and comfort provided by the familiar physical and social environment. These anchorages are replaced by strangers to whom the patient is only one of many elements to be fitted into the routine. Hence, insofar as a person can derive strength from his normal patterns of living to face illness and the prospect of death, this potential is often lost by the patient upon admission to a hospital.

From the viewpoint of family members, the patient has been removed from his accustomed relationship to them in a familiar setting to an alien one, where family members have no defined function except that of an intrusive irrelevancy. Family members face illness and death as strangers in a hospital, where they serve no instrumental purpose, and not as a functioning unit in familiar surroundings. Thus, the family's capacity to cope with the situation is weakened by the shift from home to hospital.

In the abstract, then, home care should often be preferable to hospitalization for the incurable cancer patient. But is this also true in the concrete?

The Look

Transactions between the health care system and patients fit the classic social psychology paradigm. On the one hand, there is the health care system with its capacities and goals; on the other, there are the patient and family, both with their own problems and goals. To what extent is there likely to be a mesh, to what extent a disjunction? In the case of the incurable cancer patient, are the quality and cost of home care likely to be such that hospitalization can be viewed as unnecessary and inappropriate, not only by the health care providers but also by the patient and his family?

There is no guarantee that the answer will always or even frequently be "yes." It is quite possible that the choice, hospital or home care for the cancer patient, will reflect more a decision about what is optimal for the hospital than what is optimal for the patient and family. For example, the decision to assign a patient to home care may reflect the fact that hospitals are not oriented toward the care of incurable cancer patients. Indeed, because most hospitals are cure rather than care oriented (and cure is what patients and families want), the establishment of large, formal home care programs as an integral element in the care of incurable cancer patients might well serve as a signal to the health care system that cure is for the hospital and care is for the home. This can easily lead to home care as a dumping ground for the incurable patient; the hospital would no longer be expected even to worry about assuming responsibility.

This possibility, that home care programs will become a dumping ground rather than an improved approach to the care of incurable cancer patients, may even be a probability. Over the past 15 years, there has been increasing emphasis on community and home maintenance of the mentally retarded, the mentally ill, and the orthopedically handicapped. During this same time, studies suggested that these programs were at best ineffective and at worst disruptive for the patient, the family, and the community. The past is often the best predictor of the future, and if analogous programs for other populations have failed to achieve their proponents' goals, why should we expect this one to be different?

There is a standard answer to this question—failure was the result of a lack of commitment, specifically of a lack of the necessary resources to ensure that the program would work. Indeed, this answer occurs so frequently that it is sometimes very easy to get the impression that there have never been poor programs, only underfunded ones. Cynicism aside, it is undoubtedly true that home care of the incurable cancer patient requires resources. Neither our current values nor the structure of the modern urban and suburban family facilitate acceptance of home care or coping with the demands involved in caring for a terminal cancer patient; hence, any viable program will require new and extensive supportive services. But do we know what services will be required and how much they will cost? If, as seems to be the case, we do not know what services will be required, only that they will be costly, then home care as a major component of health care for the incurable cancer patient will represent neither an improvement for the patient nor a saving for society.

Finally, we have discussed patient and family as a unit with the same goals. But is this indeed the case? Do we know that patients want to be cared for by their families or that families want to care for the patient? Social systems exist not in a vacuum but in the context of people's values and needs. We often complain that hospitals do not want responsibility for terminal patients, and yet the patients are there. Hospitals are not full of patients because the hospital recruited them; rather patient or family pressure brought them there. The fact that people have voted for hospital rather than home care by actually choosing it raises the questions of whether home care is one of those programs that people should want but do not and whether, therefore, they should not get but will get.

Conclusion

Fads and fashions come and go in health care as elsewhere. Proposals for innovations and "improvements" emerge, become popular, are adopted, and we find ourselves back where we started from. Just because home care is an idea whose time may have come is no reason to see it as a panacea or even as a plus. Until we know whether or not home care is an acceptable alternative to patients and to their families, how home care programs relate to hospital care, what supportive services are necessary and what these services cost, we should look at home care as a possibility to be explored, not as an alternative to be urged.

꩜꩜꩜ **29**

Long-Term Severe Disability

Robert Morris

A large and growing number of people now live for many years—fifteen, or even fifty years—with such severe disabilities that they require constant attention from others. In a sense one might say that the people in this group live throughout a long life confronted daily by the expectation of death and that, by and large, our present approaches for caring for them condemn them to facing this situation alone.

There is the reported case of a 50-year-old mother and her spastic adult son, both of whom had been found in their home, malnourished and enfeebled, although they had an adequate income. They had lived in this home for at least 10 years, and it is obvious that no one knew about them. They were discovered and were removed to a hospital, where a serious effort was made to keep them alive. This is not an atypical situation. There are hundreds of thousands of people across the country, I suspect, who live under such conditions.

Our attention, either to the last days of life or to making people whole again, has led to an avoidance of this group of disabled people—they number probably from 6 to 10 million people. In part, their status is the responsibility of health care professionals and not

237

something we can shift on to "society"—that vague, amoral "something" outside of ourselves. In our professions—and I include those individuals in social work, nursing, physical therapy, occupational therapy, and medicine—we have spent much time equipping ourselves to do a clean, white-collar, professional job, and we continue to prefer doing the things for which we are equipped. However, that very preparation ill equips any of us for a proper examination of the problems of long-term disability.

The Longitudinal Nature of Disability

We do not have a generic approach to the subject of severe disability, and we do not look at it in the aggregate—at the sum total of people who are confronting life-and-death problems. As professionals, we have become too highly specialized. Most of the time, when we talk about disability, we begin thinking about older people, and that is proper because they do represent a part of the problem. I would only note that for older people the problem of chronic disability and increasing enfeeblement may encumber about 20 percent of the entire lifespan. How do we deal with this? The focus is not just age but life.

But old age is only half the problem. There is ample evidence that our capacity to save the lives of infants who are born with life-threatening situations—very low birth weight, severe respiratory distress, and so on—in itself produces an increase in the proportion of persons who need the kind of attention we ought to be talking about. These very infants will grow to adulthood and will live long but disabled lives. Some studies indicate that from 6 to 15 percent of these individuals will survive with central nervous system defects that will be with them throughout life. No one knows, in an overall sense, what this adds up to, how long such children are going to live with disability, and how severe it will be.

We are able to keep alive teenagers and young adults who have had their spinal cords severed and are paralyzed from the neck or the waist down as a result of war injuries, automobile accidents, or recreational mishaps. Not many years ago, their life expectancy was a year. Now, many such young people can live 20 or 30 years, and they can lead fairly normal lives, provided there is a kind of home support system that can be the foundation on which all our highly professionalized services of medical therapy and occupational therapy and counseling are based.

If we put all of these groups together—infants, young adults, the aged—they constitute an aggregate that tells us only one thing: our great scientific advances are producing an increase in problems, not a decrease. The time is close upon us when we are going to have to give as much attention to the problems that our medicine and health care produce as we do to the support of the health system itself.

Other questions can be raised, such as "What do you do when the doctor leaves or when the hospital is not appropriate?" I emphasize this dimension because probably 95 percent of our public policy, our personnel effort, and our financing go to support medical therapy and the hospital, with little else left over for anything else. What is left over is frequently for home health services but not for home *care* services, and the distinction is important to bear in mind.

Care as a Basis for Quality of Life

If we are going to take this situation seriously, then the stance of our combined medical health and welfare professions and institutions has to be altered. We are going to have to give more thought to what is the important base for these health-welfare-medical systems to operate from. Who are significant members of the team? Although an ardent devotee of the team, I am also reminded frequently that a team approach can make possible the passing of the buck of responsibility from one member to the other. I am impressed that most discussions begin by emphasizing the kinds of things the doctor, nurse, social worker, and therapist can contribute to team operations. We then come to the home health aide or maybe a highly skilled homemaker, but we do not give much attention to the people who really make most of the difference in the lives of the people we are talking about. These are the relatively untrained people—babysitters, or friends, or homehelps, or skilled homemakers who are going to be in the household without health training but who provide physical and personal care on a day-by-day basis for a very long time.

We may have to recast our evaluation of what really is important in the lives of the disabled. Is it sufficient to concentrate as much as we do on our having a sensitive understanding and developing a relationship? I would suggest that those who make the most difference in the lives of the people we are talking about are those others who are going to be there doing home-related tasks.

These are the things that do make it bearable and possible for a family or for an individual to continue to function with the disabilities we are speaking of; lacking these, no amount of counseling, advice, and professional people to sort out priorities is going to make much difference. We need to give much more attention to what the support system really is based on, and that is attention, not necessarily at the highest therapeutic skill level, based on day-by-day helpfulness for the duration of the disability and the living part-death.

Family Versus Social Responsibility

Another dimension of the problem of long-term disability concerns the family. It is conventional for those who have followed the history of home health care programs and of home care programs based in hospitals to emphasize the importance of the family. This is essential, but it is not good enough. We are going to have to find a new balance between what we reasonably expect of a family and what our social provision is going to give to family members to help them carry on.

Examples can be cited of why this reordering of our emphasis is necessary. The capacity of a family network to care for its disabled members—even to give counseling and encouragement—is diminished very seriously in modern society, not because the family is less interested or concerned, but because of basic social changes that have taken place. We have smaller families, which means that, for many decades, we have been producing smaller family networks, that is, fewer adult children, fewer aunts, cousins, and uncles who make up the kith-and-kin network on which a disabled person can rely and on which the health care system can rely. This network is reduced by the sheer demography of our population. Families are simply smaller.

As our population ages, there is a tendency for more people to survive into their 80s and 90s and 100s, outliving their other family members and their peers. Then they have no one else remaining to look after them. (I would add that we may have an increasing proportion of our population who never create families or a viable family network because they remain single or their marriage breaks up.)

Finally, in almost all families today there is an effort on the part of all able-bodied adults, including teenaged children, to go out and work. Who is left at home to look after a disabled member, since our society and our economy seek to encourage all adult members to go out and work?

A serious reexamination is necessary of the extent to which we can proceed as professionals on the assumption that the family will always pick up the load. Families may be eager and willing to pitch in and help. But for 80 percent of the population we are talking of—the severely disabled who are discharged from medical institutions to their own homes where there is prescribed a set of home care services that include the homely sort of jobs—the families did *all* of the caring. Social provision in the form of social agencies or health agencies as a contributing partner exists in only 10 percent of the cases. At the first discharge, families were willing to pick up that load, but when there was long continuation of the need and a second hospitalization, the family's ability and willingness to carry the load alone dropped by 50 percent. I suspect that if we looked into the third and fourth hospitalization, family capacity would drop further.

We will be forced to examine what we really mean by social provision to help families "carry the load." It is just not possible to assume that we can help families sort out their priorities and face the problems of coping without, in a new dimension, supplementing their capacity to carry on. What that supplement, by social provision, will consist of has yet to be shaped, but it is obviously necessary for sick, dying, or living disabled persons who have families and for whom we want to maintain a little bit of that family care. It is even more necessary for those who do not have a family and whom we do not want to place in institutions.

Financing Long-Term Care

Aside from reexamining this relationship between social provision and the family, there are other considerations. One is obviously a change in financing, and this cannot be fantasized as a continuation of the present level of support with, by some miracle, an additional sum of money produced to pay for other things that address our attention. If we are really to grasp this nettle of disability and long-term need for help, some redistribution is going to be necessary between the amount of financing we now give (95 percent is my estimate) to hospital and medical services and the resources we allocate to necessary supplemental supportive caring services.

No easy remedy has yet been hypothesized for accomplishing this, but attention must be given to bring it about. There is some evidence that the kinds of homely home care we are speaking about can be ensured. We can identify the population at risk. We can identify the number who are going to use the service so that we have some indication about what the package of services might be and what they cost. If we are going to ensure, it makes sense only if professionals agree that it is as important to ensure these homely, relatively low-skill, low-technology services at the same level of security as we now have for those services secured by Medicare and health insurance. Whether we can strike that proper balance remains to be seen.

Agency Readiness To Deliver Long-Term Care

Finally, there must be a shift in what provider agencies are willing to take on. Most agencies in this field do a superb job. However, they have a view that the task is relatively short term, that there will be a turnover in their case loads, that they can help families pick up the load, and so forth. It is less clear whether enough of our present provider agencies are prepared to offer this other complex of services for a period of years. If our present agencies are not willing to take on the long-term task of accumulating case loads, then we will have to create a new set of provider agencies, and this prospect is linked, obviously, with the nature of our financing.

Hopeful Signs of the Future

There is a note of some hopefulness. There is a movement of two kinds in this direction. Some of it is taking place in New York City and elsewhere. The first kind is at the experimental level, a willingness to consider whether our large, permanent funding sources for medical services can be used for low-technology purposes. I refer to Medicare and Medicaid, each of which is now funding very significant substantial experiments using Medicare trust funds, in one case for older persons who are eligible for Medicare and, in the case of Medicaid, for people of low income, regardless of age.

For the first time these experiments are tapping into medical dollars to pay for social care in cases of disability, as well as for medical treatment. In some cases these experiments pay a family member to do the home caring job of the kind we are talking about; in some cases they pay a neighbor; in some cases they pay for home help, not a home health aide.

The outcome of these experiments is uncertain. They have been in operation only for a year or two, and it remains to be seen whether the evidence will indicate that the price of these kinds of service is bearable or whether we can work out a reasonable distribution of the medical care dollar. Both of these sets of experiments are premised on the assumption that the kind of home care we are talking of is a proper part of the health agencies. Just how we are going to draw the line between health and welfare may rest on the outcome of these experiments.

The second encouraging set of developments is that, frequently, without very much tax help, there is evolving around the country a small network of provider agencies sometimes connected with health, sometimes not, wherein the agencies are really taking a generic approach. They are beginning to provide under *one administrative umbrella* the whole range of services that the severely disabled may need—ranging from treatment in the hospital to physical therapy and low-skill help services at home. No longer, in these places is it necessary for one agency to do one piece of a job—to develop a relationship, to do a diagnosis, to do an assessment, to do some physical therapy, and then to refer to another agency to do all the other things, which in the end may be more vital to the quality of a life. One agency is now capable of delivering the whole range.

These programs are sometimes under state welfare auspices. Sometimes they are completely funded by private philanthropy, and sometimes they are provided for by mental health dollars or by other kinds of health dollars. They do exist. All of them are insecure. The question of whether they will survive or die on the vine depends on our assessment of what is really important, of what the priorities are for supporting a quality in life—not only the life of the person rapidly approaching death, but also the life of the person who is destined to live for a very long time with a very severe disability and who cannot function without the help of another person.

≋≋≋ Part V

Research Needs

༄༄༄ 30

Evaluation of Home Care for the Terminal Cancer Patient: A Proposed Model

Catherine Kaylor

This article describes a methodology that is relevant for the evaluation of care of the terminal cancer patient. Evaluation implies a value judgment about what is good or bad. What constitutes a quality of life for such a patient? What are the components of this quality of life? Can it be described in such a way to make measurement of success or failure possible? Definition of high-quality standards for terminal home care is the question addressed because this step precedes all others.

A brief introduction to the cancer rehabilitation and continuing care project, a three-year contract awarded the Medical College of Virginia–Virginia Commonwealth University (MCV/VCU) Cancer Center by the National Cancer Institute (NCI), is presented. Organization, services, and the plan for evaluation are described.

This project was supported by the National Cancer Institute of DHEW, Contract N01-CN-65287. Principal Investigator: Susan J. Mellette, M.D. Co-Investigator: Ernest Griffith, M.D. Evaluator: Ed Deeples, Ph.D.

A proposed systems model for evaluation of this home care program is described, with critical variables, outcomes, measures, and the overall scheme for presentation delineated. An attempt is made to define the elusive variable "quality of life" in terms of critical social, physical, and psychological functions. Data are not presented in this paper, for the purpose is chiefly to describe the rationale behind selection of critical functional variables as quality standards.

The Setting

In June 1974 the NCI awarded the MCV/VCU cancer center a three-year contract entitled "Development and Utilization of Rehabilitation and Continuing Care Resources for Cancer Patients."

Goals

Purposes of the contract were fivefold:

1. Survey needs of cancer patients.
2. Survey resources available for cancer patients.
3. Develop a program for needed clinic and at-home services using a team approach.
4. Conduct educational programs aimed at cancer care practitioners.
5. Evaluate the effects of the program.

Teams

Six cancer teams meet regularly to plan and review needs of about 300 patients monthly. The teams are composed of staff from the in-patient units, the clinics, and home care personnel paid for by the project.

Each team has a distinctive composition according to the needs of the patients it serves. The teams include head and neck, breast, gastrointestinal, pediatrics, and two continuing care teams. The two continuing care teams are for patients whose disease has spread and who usually are receiving radiation or chemotherapy. The others are teams aimed toward rehabilitation of patients who are treated for cure or control of disease.

Home Care

Not every patient is served at home, and many do not need to be seen at home. Each team averages about ten patients monthly who receive home services. However, the focus of all activity, whether in-hospital discharge planning or clinic treatment, is toward better home management of care. For the terminal patient, examples of basic at-home needs we address include evaluation for specific needs, education regarding special care, supportive counseling, assistance with finances and health coverage, maintenance of maximum physical and social function, transportation, equipment and supplies, homemaking assistance, and planning for the future of the family. Various resources are available through the project to meet these needs either directly or through coordination with community resources.

The project has provided for five nursing personnel at various levels—physical therapy, occupational therapy, speech therapy, dental hygiene, patient counseling, rehabilitation counseling, and recreation therapy. Although each staff member and an aide relate primarily to one team, they are available to patients of all teams as need and time dictate.

Methodology for Evaluation

The System
Fulfillment of the first stages of our project did not present unusual problems; however, methodology for evaluation has required a great deal of thought. Using a systems approach has helped us identify and place the elements of our program in their proper perspective and relation to one another. Crucial to this approach is a specific definition of desired outcome or quality standards on which the system

rests. Outcome definitions for our rehabilitatable patients are relatively simple. It is possible to count the number of patients who go back to work as one indicator. For other patients, work is not an appropriate goal. Outcome definitions for our continuing care of terminal patients have been difficult to arrive at because the real goal is an improved quality of life, a most elusive variable to measure.

Outcome, once defined, paves the way for answers to other questions: Which patients should be served? What services should be provided? How will one know if and when success is achieved? Figure 30.1 illustrates the elements and their relationship to each other. Each item is linked to the other, which implies that a change in one element will cause further adjustments in the system. A change in criteria of selection, an input element, can affect ultimate outcome. The feedback loop is critical for identifying potential areas needing change. For example, the definition of desired outcome may be too unrealistic and should be adjusted. It is important to measure success, but it is important to study failure as well.

Rationale
One might well ask what this has to contribute to home care of the terminal patient. Chiefly, it is an attempt to describe and quantify what happens to our patients. It is not entirely satisfactory, for some variables will be missed, and some are not capable of quantification. However, a beginning must be made. With increased possibilities for federal funding and third-party payment it becomes imperative for administrators of such programs to document what happens, why, and what the relative cost-effectiveness is of various alternatives. Improving quality of life is a worthy objective, but the commitment of dollars necessitates some attempt to determine what that quality of life consists of and whether intervention is warranted based on a cost analysis.

The question arises, why spend money on the dying when there are other pressing social needs? The answer is obvious to those who care for the dying patient. The dying patient is a living person until he draws his last breath. His concerns about a high quality of life are similar to those of other patients. He wants to preserve his independence and dignity, to remain in his own home to enjoy the support of

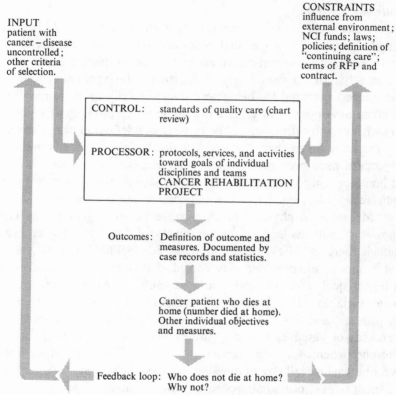

INPUT
patient with
cancer – disease
uncontrolled;
other criteria
of selection.

CONSTRAINTS
influence from
external environment;
NCI funds; laws;
policies; definition of
"continuing care";
terms of RFP and
contract.

CONTROL: standards of quality care (chart review)

PROCESSOR: protocols, services, and activities toward goals of individual disciplines and teams
CANCER REHABILITATION PROJECT

Outcomes: Definition of outcome and measures. Documented by case records and statistics.

Cancer patient who dies at home (number died at home). Other individual objectives and measures.

Feedback loop: Who does not die at home? Why not?

Figure 30.1. Evaluation Model, Cancer Rehabilitation and Continuing Care.

his family and friends, and to continue with his usual lifestyle as long as possible.

We have endless case data that must somehow be organized to demonstrate to us, funding sources, and other skeptics that we are indeed making a difference in delivery of costly services to this patient group. Regardless of the conviction we may feel as clinicians, we must have a reply to the question: How do you know? The practitioner can respond from his personal experience. However, memory is selective and arguments reduce it to "I believe." Therefore, the tremendous task of establishing objective criteria will considerably aid in reporting program effects.

Outcome Criteria

Development of outcome criteria for continuing care has been a
lengthy process, for it was first necessary to describe what needs actually exist by a comprehensive assessment of our patient population.
Ultimately, criteria should help us determine which patients will have
the greatest potential for being served successfully in the home. The
ongoing development of criteria is a complicated problem of specify-
ing what our objectives should be or what our definition of success is.
By the same token, what measures will effectively show us that our
objectives have been met? Counting the number of patients who die
at home or comparing length of hospital stay does not seem entirely
satisfactory when quality of life and comfort are the real aims.

Measures of physical function are a possible tool if they can
show that patients stay at higher levels of function longer, even
though there is an eventual and expected decline. Time of survival is another element one may consider. It is often associated with
a higher quality of life and would be useful to examine as one of
many variables. This implies the need to match with a similar group
of patients, and this may be a difficult task. Furthermore, there are
hundreds of variables that may in any one case be a critical factor.
For one patient, a critical measure of "success" was his move from
wearing pajamas all day to dressing in street clothes. Success is made
of small things, often not apparent to the evaluator.

Quality of Life

A high quality of life is an outcome that obviously is desirable for the
terminal patient. What are its components? Can it be rated in such a
way to make measurement possible? Can success or failure be as simply determined as for rehabilitation? Vocational rehabilitation defines
success as placement of a client in a job for 60 days. For continuing
care, it is a more complex issue but not impossible if one is willing to
forfeit measurement of every potential variable and select a few critical outcomes. This is often not a simple decision, as illustrated by the
patient who began wearing street clothes. In his case this was a critical variable. Professionals do not always agree. However, through
analysis of two years of case data relating to terminal care we have
decided that a high quality of life can be defined in terms of several

characteristics related to the ability to function. This does imply a value judgment on our part, but behavior and performance are more readily observed and measured. Rather than pursue philosophical issues, we define high quality of life arbitrarily and, for our purposes, include the following components: The patient is maintained in his own environment. He survives longer than a control population. His physical function is increased to the highest level possible and then maintained for as long as possible before an expected eventual decline. He is able to care for his own needs. He can manage his own care primarily in the home and does not require long hospitalization. He and his family express a reasonable sense of comfort and ability to handle stress. Community resources are used when appropriate. The patient continues with his normal level of social activity and lifestyle. The patient experiences a reasonable amount of physical comfort through treatment and prevention of complications.

Measures

After arbitrarily defining these variables we can proceed to quantify them. Some measures are frequently available in case records, such as dates of diagnosis, death, location of death, hospital admission dates, and other information (see Table 30.1).

For the remaining variables, a search was made among social psychology, sociology, and rehabilitation literature. Our need was to develop measures that practitioners could apply easily and on which judgments could be made. The measures had to fit our current data collection system and require minimal orientation in their use. Because of the need to define variables specifically in relation to a disabled or terminal cancer population, we decided to devise and adapt our own measures. The measures themselves will need further study for validation, and so initial experience with them is tentative. However, none depart radically from other measures already in existence.

Variables relating to function or behavior of the patient appear to be measurable on simple scales ranging from independent to totally dependent, with intermediate stages described. We defined these levels for several variables: physical function, including speech, ambulation, appearance, endurance and strength, self-care; social activ-

Table 30.1. Function and Behavior Scales

Ambulation

1. Independent without help
2. Independent with prosthesis or other corrective device
3. Potentially independent but needs instruction and/or encouragement
4. Minimum help of someone needed
5. Maximum help of someone needed
6. Unable to do at all
8. Not applicable
9. No response

Activity Status

1. Socially involved in activities that involve meeting new people
2. Involved in active diversion; gets out frequently
3. Interacts chiefly with family and friends; gets out occasionally; some active diversions
4. Stays primarily at home; household and yard activities, interacts mostly with family.
5. Solitary activity: passive hobbies, little interaction with others, TV, radio
6. Withdrawn, does little, socially isolated
8. Not applicable
9. No response

Self-Care

1. Independent without help
2. Independent with prosthesis or other corrective device
3. Potentially independent but needs instruction and/or encouragement
4. Minimum help of someone needed
5. Maximum help of someone needed
6. Unable to do at all
8. Not applicable
9. No response

Family Adjustment Scale

1. Well adjusted: exhibits support for patient and each other
2. Exhibits signs of some stress but still generally supportive
3. Signs of crisis: situational related primarily to illness
4. Signs of crisis: related to other family problems such as alcoholism
5. Family extremely dysfunctional: members barely able to cooperate
6. No family willing or able to help: relatives dead, institutionalized
8. Not applicable
9. No response

Emotional Adjustment

1. Patient is well adjusted
2. Patient exhibits signs of some stress but is generally adjusted
3. Patient exhibits signs of crisis: situational related to cancer
4. Patient exhibits signs of crisis: related to other problems
5. Patient is extremely dysfunctional

6. Patient is extremely dysfunctional; threat to himself or others; needs protective intervention
8. Not applicable
9. No response

Endurance and Strength

1. Sustained activity for 8 hours or more
2. Sustained activity for 4–8 hours
3. Activity 4 hours with rest periods
4. In bed 50 percent of time and up in chair only
5. In bed more than 50 percent of time but less than 100 percent
6. In bed 100 percent of time
8. Not applicable
9. No response

ity; work status; emotional status; and family adjustment status. Some of the scales are shown in Table 30.1. They were developed by a special committee and by the practitioners who will use them.

It is now possible to describe a patient's status on any one of these scales at any specific time. Correlations may also be done on the assumption that higher function should result in fewer hospital admissions. Progress of the patient can be charted over time from any appropriate point. Basically, premorbid ratings (prior to diagnosis), intake ratings (vary according to when collected), goals (highest levels achievable), and interim ratings can be collected for comparison with the status rating at closure. For example, the functional history of a patient on a particular scale might be as follows: Premorbid 1, intake 5, goal 3. Monthly interval levels of 5,5,4,3,3,5,5,6; and closing—death. So this patient reached his goal of level 3 and was maintained there for two months.

Essentially, the "best" quality of life can now be defined quantitatively as a rating on our function scales at the highest level, 1. The patient's function rating can be compared to that ideal, to the premorbid level, or to some predetermined goal based on reasonable expectation. The critical time variable of how long this high function was maintained can be determined. Goal is defined as the best potential function we can hope to reach with a given patient. For continuing care patients, this means the peak level of function and the length of time kept there. For many of these patients closing status is death. Likewise, a comparison with rehabilitatable patients will be possible by using the same scales. Difference will be accounted for by setting different goals.

Table 30.2 summarizes some of the proposed outcomes and measures.

This simplistic approach does not account for all the possible intervening variables, nor should it do so. Unexpected variance on the different scales, correlations among them, and other analyses should provide valuable clues leading to other factors that should be consid-

Table 30.2. Proposed Outcomes and Measures

Step one: Definition of desired outcome	Step two: How do you know?	Step three: Collection of data
Desired outcomes: Quality standards	Measures:	Where collected: The audit
Patient is able to die at home	Numerical count of patients who die at home	Monthly caseload reports; case record audit
Length of survival is longer than that of a control population	Compare with tumor registry data on date of diagnosis and date of death on patients with comparable diagnosis, age, disease status	Case record and tumor registry audit
Patient's level of physical function is increased to a high level and then maintained as long as possible before an eventual expected decline (includes speech, ambulation, and endurance)	Use of physical function scales and measure of time intervals patient is kept at the highest level. Time variable is critical	Monthly caseload reports; case record audit
Patient demonstrates the ability to manage his self-care	Self-care scale, which ranges from totally dependent to totally independent	Monthly caseload reports; case record audit
Patient has used hospital and clinic facilities appropriately (less often)	Hospital admission dates; unscheduled trips to clinics or ER decrease	Hospital medical record; medical oncology admission statistics
Patient and family demonstrate a reasonable sense of psychological comfort and ability to handle stress	Scales of family adjustment and patient adjustment	Monthly caseload reports; case record audit
Use of appropriate community resources	Project statistics on totals of referrals and resources used	Monthly caseload reports; case record

Table 30.2. (*Continued*)

Patient exhibits a reasonable level of socialization and activity as close to premorbid as possible	Activity rating from withdrawn and socially isolated to socially active and meeting new people	Monthly caseload reports; case record
Patient has avoided certain complications that are preventable, such as decubiti or hypercalcemia (comfort variable)	Statistics: services provided for preventable conditions and a numerical count	Case record; monthly caseload reports
	Comparison of measures over time to show times of improvement: intake, peak, interim, closing, as compared with premorbid or specified goal	
	Retrospective study to show what occurred prior to the project through tumor registry data and chart analysis	
	Comparisons of populations that currently exist but do not receive intervention merely due to caseload constraints	

Step four: Analysis 1

Step five: Feedback: How did we do?

Step six: Needed alterations in the system
 Criteria of selection
 Adjustments in services
 Data to support change of law, policies

ered. Our hope and expectation are, of course, that our intervention will make a difference. However, a description of what happens to patients can still be valuable for establishing norms. Obviously, our definition of a high quality of life is biased toward ability and duration of function. We have not attempted to rate metaphysical concerns on a scale of one to six but leave that task to theologians and philosophers.

Figure 30.1 shows how data obtained may be fed back into the system to support any needed changes in criteria of selection, adjustments in services, or policies affecting care for the terminal patient at home. Is dying at home an appropriate goal for patients? What services seem associated with "successful" outcomes? Which patients seem to fare better? Answers to these questions would be most useful to administrators dealing with decisions about program design, allocation of resources, and so forth.

Summary

An approach to evaluation of clinical practice in home care of the terminal patient that rests primarily on a definition of desired outcomes has been presented. These outcomes for the terminal patient were defined primarily in terms of specific functions and length of time maintained at the highest level. Measures were then designed on simple scales, rating the variable from highest to lowest.

Success can be defined as how closely the closing status resembles the optimum rating of one, how closely it comes to meeting a present goal, and how long the highest rating is maintained. Ability to function independently for X months becomes our major criterion against which quality of life for the terminal patient is measured on numerous variables.

In addition, practitioners may receive some feedback regarding their own efficacy. These judgments are made daily. Our plan merely attempts to assign a numerical rating to reports of success, failure, or improvement. Practitioners of many disciplines report on caseloads, including number of contacts and types of services provided for accountability to hospitals or others. With the addition of specified outcomes, goals, and measures, these monthly reports could become valuable sources of material for evaluation for the practitioner and for the field in general.

Quality assurance and professional standards review are forcing examination of outcome criteria and development of measurement tools. For the clinical practitioner the use of numbers to describe quality of life may lack appeal. However, the need to justify future funding may motivate such evaluation when generalized appeals for improving care are not sufficient.

References

Instruction for Reporting System, Division of Social Work, University of Virginia Medical Center, January 1974.

Miller, D. C. 1970. *Handbook of Research Design and Social Measurement* (2nd ed.). New York: McKay.

Rehabilitation of Cancer Patients: Final Report, Project Number RD2311-M, January 1971, Division of Research and Demonstration Grants, Social and Rehabilitation Service, Department of Health, Education and Welfare.

Statistical Reporting System, Virginia Department of Vocational Rehabilitation, Rehabilition Services Manual, July 1974.

꩜꩜꩜ Part VI
From Life to Death

≈≈≈ 31

From Life to Death

Josephine A. Lockwood

The medical literature has been replete with publications concerning "the dying patient." Of late one is impressed with the numerous seminars that have been held in many, if not most, major teaching centers and that focus on "the dying patient." Each publication and each seminar attempts to bring greater understanding of the psychological problems with which patients are confronted as they face each day in the process of life extension to the point of death. After having attended many such symposia and after having read extensively about management of families and patients termed "dying," it has been my overall impression that this total concept is counter-life thinking. The processes and dynamics pointed out are those of stepwise adjustments to life rather than to death. The reality is that these adjustments occur at a time when life expectancy is limited and, therefore, the patient's "time clock" requires resetting, as do the goals, expectations, and "time clock" of medical and paramedical staff. I think it can be readily accepted that a patient is truly "dying" in the context in which this expression is usually used if that patient is comatose or totally withdrawn and unable to respond to the surrounding environment. Dying in itself can be thought of only as a process and a continuum. It has been stated that the onset of dying begins at the moment that growth ceases; this would place that time period in adolescence. Needless to say, one's everyday experiences are not spent thinking about the shortening of life by each day lived. Rather, one would hope that each day would be accepted as life per se with inner development, a consequence of the acceptance of that life throughout its span up to and through those phases of chronic illness that will ultimately lead to death.

It has been stated, "He who fears the experience of dying is unprepared for the process of living." In so thinking, one accepts as part of life the concept of death. One incorporates all phases into one's own being and thereby potentiates greater insights into the real meaning of each moment's relationships and experiences. If one thinks in terms of dying patients, one's tendency, while attempting to explain medical care fully to all patients, is to transmit an attitude of despair to a patient undergoing such an experience. At no time, except when patients are comatose, is any patient without hope, nor should any medical staff person be without hope. The phrase "dying patient" suggests that analogy may be made to an oft-quoted phrase, "all hope abandon, ye who enter here." I would like, therefore, to turn our attention to living patients in the process of dying. Such a process may span over 30 years or three hours. In each situation those who have contact with the patient are capable of bringing renewal of hope in that moment of experience together. This is not to say that one denies the existence of serious illness and life-threatening situations but that one realistically approaches them *with the patient* and deals with the patient directly. That moment's experience represents a "life-time" experience in that very moment. Reality must be part of life experience, and preparation for tomorrow, the next month, the next year, or the next 10 years and must be ongoing. The greatest development in this area will be internal development with which the patient can be helped by the understanding of medical care personnel.

Adriaan Verwoerdt, in *Clinical Geropsychiatry* (1976), has noted that "a number of aged individuals tend to withdraw from reality and to retreat into their inner selves in order to live off their memories. A withdrawal into fantasy is the final outcome of a long process—a process which frequently begins with the experience of significant losses." The fact that such occurrences are noted in aged and chronically ill individuals is an indication that external stimuli, the multiple losses that these patients undergo, and their insecurity concerning their acceptance by neighbors, relatives, and medical staff, create these withdrawals and regression. The ultimate end to this withdrawal would be termed "advanced senile regression." Such a situation would once more represent death but in a patient who continues to have life processes working. That such a thing can happen is a reflection of the society in which we live or the manner in which we care for the elderly and chronically ill.

We might define the stages of living as follows (1) from birth to adolescence, (2) from adolescence to "adult," (3) adult living to death. Reviewing each of these three phases, one can note that, if we were to plot the total process, we would be put on an upswinging line for stage one (representing birth to adolescence, physical growth). For phase two we might indicate a plateau or cessation of physical growth, that is, maintenance and stability. For stage three we might represent a slope downward. When further analyzed, the three stages examined from the *inner-growth* aspects (i.e., the psychological development of the individual) appear entirely different. Stage one would represent some upswing; stage two, a more marked upswing; and stage three, a significantly more marked upswing. It is clear that the more experiences one incorporates into one's life, the more meaningful that life will become, and the more one will contribute to other individuals and to society as a whole.

Life—a Total Continuum

By thinking of patients in all phases of life as living patients in the process of dying, regardless of the degree and rapidity of advance of disease, we conceptually can bring about the following:

1. Continuing hope with reinforcement day by day.
2. Acceptance of naturally occurring physical and psychological events, fear being thereby diminished and enjoyment of each day's life experience being allowed.
3. Professional attitudinal changes so that patients are treated with hope and dignity and without fear on the part of professional staff in forming rela-

tionships, despite the personal threat to them at the loss of the patient cared for.

4. Family attitudes and ability to work with, and relate to, the patient's will to be enhanced. Fears will be allayed. It will become clear that there is nothing ominous about the process of aging and about the degenerative processes associated with chronic disease entities.

5. Patients' attitudes will also be changed so as not to fear rejection, suffering, and isolation. Patients will be able to continue to bring positive forces to their immediate and adjacent environments. They will think of themselves as alive and vital to all those with whom they come into contact.

In each situation in which a patient is felt to be "a dying patient," I have observed fears and changes in attitude to the detriment of the patient on the part of the patient, family, professional staff, and friends.

Summary

"What are you? I am old." A booklet published by the State Communities and Aide Association bears this title. It indicates that the question asked of so many, "What are you?" "Who are you?" can be answered in a multiplicity of ways. One will say, "I am a salesman," another, "I am a housewife," still another, "I am an artist," yet another, "I am a bank teller," and still another, "I am old." In the mind of that patient is the fear that just ahead lies the label "senile." The booklet notes that "senility is an invention of modern Western society and is one of the most damaging self-fulfilling prophecies ever devised. There is evidence that senility is much more "a functional withdrawal from painful experiences than the result of physical deterioration." Reality has little to do with the attitude that thereby arises. Social situations, lack of employment, physical disability, and isolation add to introversion. In a sense, the attitude that engenders the concept of "the dying patient" is comparable to this. It is uncomfortable for staff, friends, and families to care for "dying patient." There is, however, no discomfort in caring for living patients who at some point in time will die. That reality has been accepted consciously. This statement therefore speaks for dropping the use of language that is counter-life (i.e., referring to patients as "dying") and rather proposes that we speak of patients as living patients with a serious illness, when appropriate. With such an attitudinal change we will find that fewer tranquilizers, sleeping medications, and the like are ordered. Those medications tend to make patients fit into an already preprophesized "senile state." They are designed to "make patients manageable." That could be more easily accomplished by encouraging relationships and by bring external stimuli to the patient. If our society were comparable to those of several areas within the world where life and productive living continue past the age of 100, if patients were able to bring their experiences to others and to continue working and have continued involvement, senility and dying without dignity might come to an end.

Reference

Verwoerdt, A. 1976. *Clinical Geropsychiatry.* Baltimore: Williams and Wilkins.

꧁꧁꧁ 32

Connotations of Hospitalization

Susan J. Mellette

The emotional connotations hospitalization has for patients may be derived from a vast array of factors ranging from hearsay to the experiences of themselves or of friends. For some, especially the elderly, the centuries-old concept of a hospital as a "place to die" still lingers. For others, the image of a hospital may be derived from television depictions of places in which all sorts of new and near miraculous operations are performed and cures effected. Cancer patients who know or suspect the nature of their disease may be particularly susceptible to such a hope; and indeed, in many cases it is a justified one.

Some may almost welcome the prospect of hospitalization, because the hospital represents a place where they will be coddled and cared for as individuals. Previous hospitalizations may have pleasant connotations for some: Women whose only prior experience with a hospital has been on the maternity floor may well have forgotten the delivery, and remember only a room full of roses and an admiring husband and family. Patients who have exhausted themselves in trying to carry on their usual activities in spite of major symptoms of disease may see the hospital as an escape—a place for respite and rest.

268

A physician's recommendation that a patient be hospitalized for cancer treatment should meet several criteria. The first is rather clear: the treatment is needed. An obvious example would be an operation, which of course requires that the patient be in a hospital where specialized equipment and staff are available. However, preliminary studies (x-rays, radioisotope scans, blood or bone marrow studies), can often be carried out on an out-patient basis, either before, or sometimes instead of, hospitalization. As the result of such a work-up, it may be concluded that radiation therapy or chemotherapy would be the most appropriate; and either of these can usually be given on an out-patient basis.

A second criterion for hospitalization should be that it represents the more effective or the safer way in which treatment can be given. It may be possible to give a course of chemotherapy on an outpatient basis; but a patient who lives a hundred miles away may not be physically able to make the necessary trips. Furthermore, the physician may find it difficult to make an adequate evaluation of the effects of the treatment, particularly during an initial course, if the patient can be seen only infrequently. Sometimes, the use of a boarding home or a hospital self-care unit may be an effective means for providing continuity of care for a patient whose home is too far away for him to commute easily for radiation therapy or intermittent courses of chemotherapy.

Case Illustration

Patient E. L., a 59-year-old male, was referred in September 1969 with a diagnosis of malignant melanoma metastatic to liver, to the extent that the liver filled practically all of the abdominal cavity. Pulmonary metastases were also present. Treatment was begun with vincristine and a nitrosourea, a plan which required injections once monthly. Because the patient lived nearly 200 miles away, and because of the experimental nature of the treatment, readmission for two or three days each month was advised and accepted. This was usually planned for a week-end in order to allow the patient to continue at his work, and an advance reservation was made at the time of each discharge. After the first six months, the initial dramatic response to treatment was diminishing, and a longer course of treatment (5 days) with imidazole carboxamide was instituted each month for two courses. Treatment with oral hydroxyurea was begun in July 1970, and arrangements made with the patient's local physician to follow the blood counts and liver chemistries. Only one evaluatory hospitalization was necessary during the following ten months, during which the patient's general condition remained stable, and telephone contact was maintained between the patient's local physician and the medical oncologist, as well as between the patient and both physicians. In the late spring of 1971, there was evidence of progressive disease, and new investigational treatments were again instituted, with two more visits to the Cancer Center during the next three months. Eventually, the condition deteriorated in spite of continued treatments, and the patient was hospitalized for terminal care in his local hospital where he died, over two years after the diagnosis of widespread metastases from malignant melanoma.

In this case, appropriate uses were made of different varieties of hospitalization and out-patient care. The local hospital was the site of the original biopsy to prove liver metastases; but the Cancer Center Hospital was used to provide specialized treatment which could not be given elsewhere. The several Center hospitalizations were to the Self-Care Unit, where the patient's wife stayed with him in a motel-type room. The duration of these stays was from two to nine days, with an average of about four days each for 11 hospitalizations over a two-year period. The patient and his wife developed a warm affection for the various members of the Center staff, and actually looked forward to the scheduled visits. However, at the terminus of his illness, the local hospital provided a more appropriate and convenient setting.

A third criterion for hospitalization involves the recognition of the previously mentioned psychological reactions to hospitalization. A patient may misinterpret the necessity for hospitalization, and become convinced that admission is being advised because of major deterioration when in fact only a treatment regime is indicated. The reasons for hospitalization must, therefore, always be explained, sometimes in detail; preferably, she should be told approximately how long she is likely to stay. Occasionally, an opposite reaction occurs at the time of discharge; the patient may decide that she is being sent home "because nothing more can be done." Again, a straightforward talk with the patient about her status and the merits of hospitalization versus outpatient care may clarify the situation.

The patient who asks to be hospitalized presents a special problem. While the reasons for such a request may be apparent, sometimes there are hidden meanings. For example, the patient may actually feel so badly that she can no longer function at home. Are other family members, for one reason or another, making her life at home unpleasant? Or is she simply trying indirectly to determine just how sick she really is? The physician who concurs with such a request simply because it is made may be missing an opportunity to determine some of the underlying, and more basic, emotional problems.

There are, however, some specific situations in which hospitalization may be advised for reasons which are other than strictly medical.

Case Illustration

Mrs. M., a 40-year-old woman with breast cancer had only recently been divorced and remarried to a man, also recently divorced. The discovery of her metastatic bone disease had come as a shock to both of them; and the husband had sobbed inconsolably when he had been told in private of his new wife's prognosis. It came as a shock, then, to the physician when the patient came in for an outpatient visit a few weeks later covered with bruises. These, she said, had been inflicted by her husband. When she returned a week later with more bruises and an increase in bone pain stated to have been secondary to his beating her, it seemed advisable to take some action. The physician admitted the patient to the Self-Care Unit, to "hide" her, and to allow a "cooling off" period. Three days later, the patient and her husband arrived hand in hand. He had found her, and they had had a "second honeymoon" in the Self Care Unit. He had gradually been able to get over his anger and the need to vent his hostility toward the disease on its victim. Over the next two years of her disease, he appeared to be the paragon of an affectionate husband. About two weeks before she died, the wife one day spontaneously brought up the incident.

"Do you remember the trouble my husband and I had a couple of years ago? Well, I just wanted to tell you there's never been anything like that again. During the past few weeks that I've been in bed or in a wheelchair, he's handled me like a baby; I just never could have made it these years without him.''

That statement coincided with the situation as we had observed it; and the physician was again glad that she had not been judgmental, that she had effectively utilized a hospitalization for meeting a need which might have been considered inappropriate by a bed-utilization committee.

⚘⚘⚘ Epilogue

Samuel Klagsbrun and Lois Jaffe

Dr. Klagsbrun:	Lois, could you tell us about yourself?
Mrs. Jaffe:	I am an acute leukemia patient and have been in my first remission for over two years.
Dr. Klagsbrun:	Time must have a very special meaning for you compared to the way you thought about time prior to your illness. The idea of not wanting to put up with any nonsense from anyone must be a very important part of your approach to people.
Mrs. Jaffe:	Yes, I have always had trouble with that. I grew up in the South where magnolias dripped with honey, and I was socialized because of my own family and cultural patterns into never saying anything unpleasant, never showing negative feelings, and never showing anger. That has been a very difficult thing for me to deal with, and I was angry as hell when I became ill. At first I had to find ways to channel that anger, like writing the hospital board and the x-ray department about how terrible their services were, complaining bitterly, and so on. I had to put it on paper and make it very rational. Little by little, I have reached the point of thinking, "What am I going to lose? What can anybody do to me?" I

273

am much freer to express anger and to express negative feelings now. I had no trouble expressing positive feelings; it is the negative feelings that scared me. The time sense has certainly done that.

Dr. Klagsbrun: In a way the obstacles that take place very often in bringing good treatment to a patient facing any kind of illness, and especially terminal illness, at the end of life become even greater. They are difficult to overcome in official institutional settings.

Regulations and certain cultures occur in places such as in a hospital. There have been some people who have tried to take the terminal patient out of the official hospital setting, or at least to create a new culture around that patient within a hospital setting. The term *hospice* has been adopted for that experience or setting, which implies caring for the patient and paying particular attention, not to the purely medical management, but to all the other aspects of life that are obviously important. How to live well until you die is what it amounts to. This includes pain management, paying attention to the family—everything possible that one can do to bring the home into the hospital or hospice setting. A prime example of this is, of course, St. Christopher's Hospice in London, England, run by Dr. Cicely Saunders, who has pioneered in this field. How much thought have you given to the time of life when your body will not respond to chemotherapy and the illness becomes increasingly progressive and encroaches on your life, a time when you will have to rely on a great deal of support from others?

Mrs. Jaffe: Obviously, I have thought about it. In the summer I want sunshine, flowers, and green grass. Physical environment is important to me because I love color and texture. I love going barefoot in the green grass. I would like to experience that. I am not con-

cerned about the social environment so much because I have a second family in the hospital. I feel
very close and intimate to the people who take care
of me medically and have no fear of abandonment
from them or my family What does frighten me is
when there are many deaths in the ward, and the
nurses share with me and other patients as well,
their sense of frustration, sadness, and rage, and
their wanting to leave. I worry and get scared when
I think that the people I've become most attached
to, such as the nurses—only they are there on a
continuing basis—may leave as many have. But I
have enough trust in the basic core that they will
remain, and I trust my doctor implicitly. So it is not
the social environment in terms of my caregivers
that bothers me. Rather, it is the fact that there is no
room for privacy; there is no room with a soft rug,
dim lights, color, and a couch that is not associated
with pain, that I can go to where I can be intimate
with my husband. There is no place I can be with
my family that is not a dismal, gray, bare room
because no money is invested in that unit where
people die. There is no lounge chair that my husband can stretch out on and spend the night with me
if I am critical. Only young people with sleeping
bags manage to do that, and I want my husband
with me. If I cannot be at home, I want a home environment so that my children will feel comfortable
coming. It is hard enough for them to confront my
death, and for me to confront it with them, aside
from battling an impersonal, bleak, dreadful physical environment. I want it to be as natural as any
other part of my life. My dying should be a part of
my life that does not seem set off and pathological
and disease ridden. Dying is a natural part of my
life. The trouble with our society is that we look at
dying as pathology and disease. My desire is to

make my dying environment as natural as possible to simulate what has been my living environment.

Dr. Klagsbrun: You have just described a marvelous hospice setting—making sure that the emphasis is on the person, and not on the management of disease, even at the end of life.

Mrs. Jaffe: My fantasy where I might spend my last days, if it cannot be at home, is to be in a room where one entire wall is glass with a sliding door. With whatever energies I have left or with help, I would want to slide that glass door open and move out into the sunshine with the flowers and the green grass. I would love to die outdoors, as a matter of fact. I love the outdoors.

Dr. Klagsbrun: Almost everyone that I have talked to or worked with in this area has different feelings. There are those people who are aware of that description as a possibility or a goal, and people who have given up because they have spent too much time in a hospital setting and surrender to it. They feel that there is no other way except that of the siderails, the oxygen tank, or outlet in the back, the incandescent light at the top, and usually either gray (there used to be a time when the color was institutional green in hospitals) or sickly blue walls.

Mrs. Jaffe I would swap for the sickly blue. When I get depressed at the hospital, I will put my clothes on and go outside to where there is a small patch of grass and sit in the sun. This is as acceptable as my breathing on that unit. I am really plugging for, and the administration is now talking about, moving the unit to another floor with more space, more privacy, and the opportunity to take a rooftop and make it into a sun roof. You are quite right. You get used to the environment that you are in. It is good and it is bad. You can tolerate what is expected and adjust yourself to what *is,* rather than keep using any energies you have to push for what you would wish. I hope as long as I have any energy left to keep pushing for what could be, and not to just accept what is.

From tapings made by Lois Jaffe for the Foundation of Thanatology at its Symposium "The Role of the Social Worker in Caring for the Dying Patient and the Family" (April 1975).

ᕫᕫᕫ Index

279

❧❧❧ List of Contributors

CHARLES ADSIT, Jr., M.D., St. Luke's Hospital Center, New York, New York

JEANNE QUINT BENOLIEL, D.N.Sc., Professor and Chairman, Department of Comparative Nursing Care Systems, School of Nursing, University of Washington, Seattle, Washington

NAOMI BLUESTONE, M.D., Coordinator, Social Medicine, Residency Program in Social Medicine, Montefiore Hospital and Medical Center, Bronx, New York

IRENE G. BUCKLEY, M.A., ACSW, CSW, Executive Director, Cancer Care, Inc. of The National Cancer Foundation, Inc., New York, New York

STANLEY BUDNER, Ph.D., Associate Professor, Center for Community Health Systems of Columbia University, New York, New York

DANIEL BURDICK, M.D., Clinical Professor of Surgery, State University of New York, Upstate Medical Center, Syracuse, New York

RICHARD CHASSÉ, M.A., Patient Counselor/Chaplain, Cancer Rehabilitation Program, Medical College of Virginia, Virginia Commonwealth University, Richmond, Virginia

ISABELLE M. CLIFFORD, M.P.H., Home Health Consultant, Private Practice, Buffalo, New York

JEAN COLLARD, M.A., Instructor in Clinical Social Work, Department of Neurology, College of Physicians and Surgeons, Columbia University; Associate Director, Social Services, Neurological Institute, Columbia-Presbyterian Medical Center, New York, New York

JOSEPHINE K. CRAYTOR, R.N., M.S., F.A.A.N., Professor Emeritus, School of Nursing, University of Rochester; Cancer Center, University of Rochester Medical School, Rochester, New York

W. A. L. LYALL, M.D., Associate Professor of Psychiatry, University of Toronto, Canada; Staff Psychiatrist, Clarke Institute of Psychiatry; Consultant, Ontario Cancer Institute, Toronto, Canada

SUSAN J. MELLETTE, M.D., Associate Professor (Medical Oncology), Medical College of Virginia, Virginia Commonwealth University, Richmond, Virginia

FLORENCE MOORE, Executive Director, National Council for Homemaker-Home Health Aid Services, Inc., New York, New York

ROBERT MORRIS, Ph.D., Kirstein Professor of Social Planning, The Florence Heller Graduate School for Advanced Studies in Social Welfare, Brandeis University, Waltham, Massachusetts

STEVEN A. MOSS, Coordinator of Jewish Chaplaincy Service, Memorial Sloan-Kettering Cancer Center, New York, New York

LEONIE NOWITZ, MSW, Social Worker, Jewish Home and Hospital for the Aged, Bronx, New York

EDITH OAKES, Coalition for Home Health Services, Syracuse, New York

H. POLLACK, Ph.D., Psychologist, Clarke Institute of Psychology, Toronto, Canada

ELIZABETH R. PRICHARD, M.S., Assistant Professor of Clinical Social Work, Department of Medicine, College of Physicians and Surgeons, Columbia University; Director, Social Services, The Presbyterian Hospital in the City of New York, Columbia-Presbyterian Medical Center, New York, New York

ISADORE ROSSMAN, M.D., Home Care, Montefiore Hospital and Medical Center, Bronx, New York

MOLLIE SCHWARTZ, Coalition for Home Health Services, Syracuse, New York

IRENE B. SEELAND, M.D., Associate in Clinical Psychiatry, Department of Psychiatry, College of Physicians and Surgeons, Columbia University, New York, New York

JANET STARR, Executive Director of The Coalition for Home Health Services in New York State, Syracuse, New York

REGINA SUGRUE, Senior Companion Program, United Neighborhood Homes of New York, Inc., New York, New York

ODESSA THOMPSON, Coalition for Home Health Services, Syracuse, New York

M. L. S. VACHON, R.N., M.A., Research Scientist, Clarke Institute of Psychiatry; Assistant Professor, Department of Psychiatry, University of Toronto; Psychiatric Nurse Consultant, Ontario Cancer Institute, Toronto, Canada

VIRGINIA G. WESSELLS, R.N., M.S.N., Medical College of Virginia, Virginia Commonwealth University, Richmond, Virginia

MARIE G. WILSON, MSW, Project Director, Senior Companion Program, United Neighborhood Houses of New York, Inc., New York, New York

SALLY WOODRING, R.N., St. Luke's Hospital Center, Women's Hospital, New York, New York

Columbia University Press / *Foundation of Thanatology Series*

Teaching Psychosocial Aspects of Patient Care
Bernard Schoenberg, Helen F. Pettit, and Arthur C. Carr, editors

Loss and Grief: Psychological Management in Medical Practice
Bernard Schoenberg, Arthur C. Carr, David Peretz, and Austin H. Kutscher, editors

Psychosocial Aspects of Terminal Care
Bernard Schoenberg, Arthur C. Carr, David Peretz, and Austin H. Kutscher, editors

Psychosocial Aspects of Cystic Fibrosis: A Model for Chronic Lung Disease
Paul R. Patterson, Carolyn R. Denning, and Austin H. Kutscher, editors

The Terminal Patient: Oral Care
Austin H. Kutscher, Bernard Schoenberg, and Arthur C. Carr, editors

Psychopharmacologic Agents for the Terminally Ill and Bereaved
Ivan K. Goldberg, Sidney Malitz, and Austin H. Kutscher, editors

Anticipatory Grief
Bernard Schoenberg, Arthur C. Carr, Austin H. Kutscher, David Peretz, and Ivan K. Goldberg, editors

Bereavement: Its Psychosocial Aspects
Bernard Schoenberg, Irwin Gerber, Alfred Wiener, Austin H. Kutscher, David Peretz, and Arthur C. Carr, editors

The Nurse as Caregiver for the Terminal Patient and His Family
Ann M. Earle, Nina T. Argondizzo, and Austin H. Kutscher, editors

Social Work with the Dying Patient and the Family
Elizabeth R. Prichard, Jean Collard, Ben A. Orcutt, Austin H. Kutscher, Irene Seeland, and Nathan Lefkowitz, editors